PRAISE FOR *SLOW MEDICINE*

"Anybody considering medical school, or already toiling there, has to read this book. Everyone else should, too. . . . [Sweet's] memoir of growing slowly into her calling is about learning not just to save lives but to make a life. . . . Her personal odyssey is more stirring than any polemical manifesto could be."

—*The Atlantic*

"Wonderful . . . often lyrical . . . subtle and insightful . . . Physicians would do well to learn this most important lesson about caring for patients from Sweet's book."

—*The New York Times Book Review*

"An impassioned plea for a more humane system of healing—and a great read for everyone involved in medicine as patient or practitioner."

—*San Francisco Chronicle*

"Through the moving stories of patients and her experiences in medical school, [Sweet] explores how she found a compassionate way to care. A thoughtful companion to one of today's hot-button issues."

—*Good Housekeeping*

"Dr. Sweet writes as if she was sitting at our kitchen table, quietly and compassionately teaching about our bodies and our lives."

—*New York Journal of Books*

"[Sweet] offers an alternative to the tyranny of efficiency at the expense of healing."

—*Good Times* (Santa Cruz)

"Beautiful . . . [Sweet's] prose is clear and direct, with a warmth and intelligence that engages the reader from the book's first pages. . . . A sober and lucid examination of what we lose when medicine is shaped by economics and not vocation, when it is informed by litigation and not reverence. One can only hope, and pray, that Sweet is not a prophet crying in the wilderness."

—*St. Cloud Visitor*

"[A] master storyteller . . . highly readable . . . the sick will take comfort in this physician's warm, personal, knowledgeable approach."

—*Kirkus Reviews*

"Profoundly intimate . . . Sweet provides a strong and necessary tonic as health care, in all its complexities, remains at the center of the national conversation."

—*Booklist*

"Sound advice that all involved in health care should heed. [*Slow Medicine*] will appeal to both professional and lay readers."

—*Library Journal*

Slow Medicine

THE WAY TO HEALING

Victoria Sweet

RIVERHEAD BOOKS

New York

RIVERHEAD BOOKS
An imprint of Penguin Random House LLC
375 Hudson Street
New York, New York 10014

The Library of Congress has catalogued the Riverhead hardcover edition as follows:

Names: Sweet, Victoria, author.
Title: Slow medicine : the way to healing / Victoria Sweet.
Description: New York : Riverhead Books, 2017.
Identifiers: LCCN 2017017463 (print) | LCCN 2017026619 (ebook) |
ISBN 9780698183711 (ebook) | ISBN 9781594633591 (hardback)
Subjects: LCSH: Medicine. | Chronically ill—Care. | Healing. | Physician and
patient. | BISAC: MEDICAL / Physician & Patient. | BIOGRAPHY &
AUTOBIOGRAPHY / Medical. | MEDICAL / Healing.
Classification: LCC RA973.5 (ebook) | LCC RA973.5 S94 2017 (print) |
DDC 610—dc23
LC record available at https://lccn.loc.gov/2017017463
p.   cm.

First Riverhead hardcover edition: October 2017
First Riverhead trade paperback edition: October 2018
Riverhead trade paperback ISBN: 9780399573316

BOOK DESIGN BY NICOLE LAROCHE

For My Teachers

Named and unnamed, known and unknown

Contents

Slow Medicine

Medicine Without a Soul

I didn't know how bad it was until my own father was in the hospital. It began on Friday afternoon of the week before Thanksgiving, not the best time to get sick. Even hospitals and doctors have a kind of schedule, and Friday afternoons are when we like to straighten things up for the weekend. My father came back from lunch at a restaurant with my mother, lay down for a rest, and then she observed him having a seizure.

This wasn't new. He'd had a few grand mal seizures over the years and was supposed to be taking seizure medication, but sometimes did not. And though my mother had seen him have seizures before, she was terrified; seizures are terrifying, though mostly they don't hurt you.

She called 911, the paramedics brought him to the lovely community hospital five blocks from their house, he was examined and admitted.

That surprised me. Where I usually practice medicine, in a public hospital in San Francisco, he would never have been admitted for a simple, recurrent grand mal seizure. We would have checked his labs and gotten a CT scan, observed him overnight in the emergency room, cranked up his seizure medication, and spit him out the next morning.

Instead, at the little community hospital, the doctors were going to take their time, get his seizure medication right, let my aged mother sleep that night. How humane.

I reassured the family. I would come up the next afternoon when he would be recovering from his post-seizure state and would doubtless be discharged. He would probably be better than he'd been before. Terrifying as they are to see, grand mal seizures clear the brain; shock therapy, which sends a jolt of electricity through the brain, is designed to do the very same thing. With a grand mal seizure, everything shuts down at once, and then, rather like rebooting a computer, the faculties come back up, one by one. First the eyes open, then the body moves, then the patient smiles. Speech comes back, then memory. In a certain way, grand mal seizures are good for you; they allow, in the same way rebooting your computer does, for everything to get reorganized, re-filed. There's a clarity afterward, a quickness; the connections are connecting right again.

But when I walked into my father's private room, with its view of the mountains, its natural light, I was shocked. He was in four-point restraints, arms and legs tied to the bed corners, and he was unconscious, with a bloody bag of urine at the foot of his bed. Mother was sitting next to him, looking frightened and gray.

They had been together by that time for sixty-eight years, in a kind of Romeo and Juliet relationship, if you can imagine how irritable Romeo would have gotten after those first twenty years, how bossy, and how stressed Juliet would have been with anything in life that upset Romeo, including herself. My mother was still beautiful, and my father still a nice-looking man. White hair, blue-gray eyes by turns attentive, skeptical, and teasing, he was careful of his appearance. Shirt and tie and jacket, and manners. He still opened doors for women and moved to the street side when you walked with him. He was always tough. Uncomplaining. I'd never seen him defeated, frightened, or cowed, until that afternoon.

I left the room to find his doctor, or, to be precise, the hospitalist assigned to him for that shift. Dr. Day was alone at the nursing station, typing into a computer. I went over and introduced myself as a physician. He was in a hurry, I could tell, with other patients waiting to be seen, a state I know well. Although he didn't turn his eyes from the screen, he did explain.

"Your father came in last night with a first-time seizure, and of course we admitted him to rule out a stroke. His first CT scan was negative, so we've scheduled him for a repeat CT tomorrow, since, as you know, sometimes the first CT after a stroke is negative."

I was taken aback. This was not Father's first seizure but simply another in a series of seizures. And the distinction was crucial, because in a man his age, a first seizure would almost certainly be from a stroke, and he would need the stroke protocol of care. On the other hand, a seizure in a person with a history of seizures means, usually, that he simply forgot to take his medication.

"But this isn't a first-time seizure," I clarified. "He's had seizures for years."

Dr. Day stopped typing. He looked puzzled. "I'm sure I saw 'first-time seizure' in his electronic health record. . . . Let me look it up. . . . Ah, yes, here it is. I thought so. The neurologist's admission note—'first-time seizure, rule out stroke.'"

"But it's not his first seizure, it's one of many. See, he even has an allergy to a seizure medication on his list of allergies, right here." I was looking at the computer screen over his shoulder and pointed it out.

"Hmmmm . . . Yes, you're right. I should change the diagnosis then."

Dr. Day spent quite a bit of time trying to change the diagnosis in the computer but did not seem satisfied with his results. "Well, we'll order another CT scan. Sometimes strokes don't show up on the first scan."

I went back into Father's room to get another look. Perhaps I was missing something. Perhaps he'd had a stroke at the exact same moment as his seizure.

Father was asleep. He was alone. There was an IV running in his arm, a catheter in his bladder, and a clip on his finger sending his blood pressure and pulse wirelessly to a computer outside. I sat down on the bed and he opened his eyes. He hadn't been sleeping but pretending to be asleep. Then I examined him for any sign of a stroke. His pupils were equal and reactive, his arms and legs were of equal strength, there was no change to his face. He was drowsy, for sure; he was still recovering from his seizure, sedated from the tranquilizer he was getting, and sleep-deprived. But that was all.

"When do I get out of here?" he asked me.

"Pretty soon. They want to do another brain scan first."

Then I went out to ask Dr. Day the reason for the catheter and the four-point restraints. He was gone. No one else was around either. Not a nurse, not a nursing assistant, not a janitor.

Father had a rocky night. He was restless and the catheter hurt him, and he kept trying to pull it out, so he was tranquilized further and kept in restraints. His second CT scan was also negative, but the stroke protocol continued nonetheless. Dr. Day's attempts to change the electronic health record diagnosis of "stroke" must have been unsuccessful. So when I visited Father the next afternoon, he was still tied up, and the catheter still in. By now his beard was growing out; he was unwashed, exhausted, puzzled, and alone. And weak. Because of the stroke diagnosis, he hadn't been given anything to eat, and he hadn't had a calorie for two days.

"How am I going to get out of here?" he asked me. "Can you spring me? They don't give me anything to eat, they've tied me up, I can't even scratch my nose."

"You'll get out of here, but it'll take a while. The main thing is, when they come in and ask you the date and the place and the president, stop telling them it's Millard Fillmore. They don't know who he is, they don't realize you're joking, and they think you're crazy."

He looked up at me, his blue eyes still capable of twinkling. "Okay."

Although, as I would see when I later went through his electronic health records, no one did come in and ask him the date, the place, or the president. Every single person—hospitalist, nurse, therapist—simply stood in the doorway, saw an old man unshaven and tied up, and checked the box labeled "Confused."

Every day he had a different hospitalist, who followed the stroke protocol, although Father hadn't had a stroke. Speech therapy came by in the morning while he was still sedated from the night's tranquilizers and determined it would be dangerous to give him anything by mouth. Physical therapy came by and determined it was dangerous for him to get out of bed. Aspirin, blood thinners, and blood pressure medicine were all started. It would have been 100 percent quality assurance, if he'd had a stroke.

Finally Thursday arrived, when the hospital would start preparing its Friday discharges, Thanksgiving notwithstanding, and that afternoon I met the first person I'd yet seen inside his room. She was also the first person wearing a white coat. She carried a clipboard and looked serious.

Father was very sick, she told me—stroke—and he wasn't allowed to have anything by mouth, so the family should begin thinking about a feeding tube. He couldn't go home, of course, and she was recommending his discharge to a rehabilitation facility . . . tomorrow.

Who was she? I wanted to know.

She was the Quality Assurance Manager, she said, putting out her hand. Glad to meet you. Your father. Stroke, so sad. She shook her head sympathetically and left.

So the next day he was discharged to the rehabilitation facility, untied, and taken off the tranquilizers. He began to wake up, walk with a walker, and eat the pureed food he was now allowed. But he still had the catheter because no one ordered it to be removed. It hurt and he wanted it out, and that Monday morning, he pulled it out himself and then collapsed.

When I saw him in the emergency room a few hours later, I gave him a fifty percent chance of surviving.

His blood pressure was very low; he was gray, barely conscious, and obviously septic with bacteria in his blood. Now he was admitted to the lower-level ICU, the SDU (Step-Down Unit) on three antibiotics, with the catheter back in, and as a patient who'd had a stroke and couldn't eat. Even though he hadn't had a stroke. No one had been able to change that initial diagnosis in the electronic health records, "first-time seizure, rule out stroke." So—nothing by mouth, saltwater in his veins, tied to the bed corners, and sedated.

Now, I have three sisters, and two of them had been keeping watch, but finally the third sister, the lawyer, flew in, took one look at him, and moved into his hospital room. That's how we learned what wasn't being done—feeding him, comforting him, changing the sheets without hurting him, not to speak of getting the right diagnosis and the right treatment.

What were we going to do?

We had a family meeting.

Things were going from bad to worse, we all agreed. We had to get Father out of the hospital as soon as possible, and sooner off the catheter, the restraints, and the tranquilizers. But how?

There was only one way, I knew, to save our father. Only one way. Hospice. We would have to convince whichever current hospitalist he had that the family had decided to let Father go. If we didn't, then the next stop on his Death Express would be a *Clostridium difficile* infection from the antibiotics he was getting for the urine infection in his blood from the catheter he didn't need, followed by a bedsore, a nursing home, and a prolonged, expensive, dwindling death.

So the next morning I tracked down his current hospitalist, who happened to be Dr. Day, his first doctor, the every-twelve-hours cycle of different physicians having come around again.

"We had a family meeting last night," I began. Hospitalists like family meetings, I knew. "We went over Father's course and we agreed: he's ninety-three; he's lived a good life; it's time. So we've decided to take him home. We'll have round-the-clock care and my sister the lawyer is talking with hospice right now."

Dr. Day looked up at me from his computer. He frowned. But he did start typing in the discharge orders. "You know, I would never do this if you weren't going to do hospice."

"Yes, of course."

"He needs two more days of IV antibiotics."

"Uh-huh."

He sighed. He didn't really believe me.

I listened to the click of the keys as he typed. How satisfying. Discontinue catheter. Discontinue restraints. Discontinue sedatives, IVs, oxygen, and pureed diet. Discharge patient.

Five hours after those clicks, Father arrived home, rolling out of the ambulance in a gurney and demanding a steak and a beer. He was hungry, he said, and they had never fed him—not once!—in that hospital. He ate the steak and drank the beer, no problem.

A few hours later, hospice arrived. They did everything the hospital didn't do. They looked at Father and touched him; they sat on his bed. They talked to Mother. They figured the family out and realized pretty quickly that Father wasn't dying anytime soon. Then they were humane and smart. They let him stay on hospice for two months, until he was recovered from his near-fatal hospital admission and back to his pre-hospital self.

"Hospice" is proof that the problem with healthcare is not in the players but in something else.

I'd known that healthcare was getting ever more bureaucratic; that doctors and nurses had less and less time to take care of their patients;

that they were spending more and more of their time in front of a computer screen entering health-care data. I'd experienced it myself. But until that week, I had no idea how bad it had become. If I, as a physician, couldn't get appropriate care for a family member in a lovely community hospital with well-trained staff—who could?

What had happened to medicine and nursing? I asked myself.

To find out, I ordered up Father's electronic health records and went over his near-death experience.

The document was 812 pages long and took me four hours to read. It began not with the doctors' notes but with hundreds of pages of pharmacy orders; then hundreds of pages of nursing notes, which were simply boxes checked. Only the doctors' notes were narrative, and mostly they were cut-and-paste. No wonder no one could figure out what was really going on. Still, to be fair, although I found mistakes in the records, Father had, after all, gotten discharged, and even if he had stayed in the hospital for those extra two days, he probably would have gotten home. Sure, he might have had a bedsore or a fall. But I had to admit, judging by those electronic health records, his stay in the hospital looked 100 percent quality-assured.

There was just something missing. And it was hard to put my finger on it.

Everything looked so good in the computer, and yet what Father had gotten was not Medicine but Healthcare—Medicine without a soul.

What do I mean by "soul"?

I mean what Father did not get.

Presence. Attention. Judgment.

Kindness.

Above all, responsibility. No one took responsibility for the story. The essence of Medicine is story—finding the right story, understanding the true story, being unsatisfied with a story that does not make sense. Healthcare, on the other hand, deconstructs story into thousands of tiny pieces—pages of boxes and check marks for which no one is responsible.

A robot doctor could have cared for my father just as well.

What happened to my father is one example of how medicine is being practiced today, or, rather, how healthcare is being provided. Not every civilization has cared about the health of its citizenry. But we do. We spend 17.5 percent of our GDP, 17.5 percent of our energy and resources, on health, sickness, and disease. And yet we've ended up with a health-care system in which the only way to get good medical care is to go home to die.

My father's hospital looked so great, with its cheerful website announcing its "dedication to treating the whole patient." Many of the staff had even read my book, *God's Hotel*. The book was about my experience being a doctor in an unusual hospital in San Francisco. I'd titled it *God's Hotel* because that's what hospitals were once called, back in the Middle Ages: *hôtels-Dieu*. The replacement of Medicine by Healthcare had come to that hospital while I was practicing there, and I'd written the book as a cautionary tale—don't let this happen to your hospital, to your doctor. Some of the staff at my father's hospital had read it at their book club, and the Chief of Medicine asked me for my autograph. And still my father could not get the kind of care at their hospital that doctors, nurses, and even marketing people know is needed.

So the experience with my father shocked me. It highlighted the difference between my own version of medicine and the version being put into place even as I write. By "version of medicine" I mean the complex of ideas that comes out of whichever model we use for the body, and the way of healing that results from that.

My own version of medicine began to form in medical school, when I learned modern medicine, which is based on the idea that the body is best understood as a machine or a collection of machines. So the brain is a computer, the heart is a pump, the lungs are bellows, the kidney a filtering device. Disease, therefore, is a breakdown, and the doctor is a mechanic whose job is to find what's broken and fix it or replace it. The way of healing that comes out of this model is focused; it is a taking apart and peering in, reductionist, linear, and step-by-step. It is a powerful way of understanding the body, the main reason for the incredible progress of modern medicine, and I use it still.

But as I began to see patients I also began to realize that there was something missing from that version of medicine. It explained a lot, but not everything—that patients sometimes get better on their own; the importance of relationship; the healing effects of time.

I looked around for another model for understanding my patient, and I found it in premodern medicine, when the body was thought to be best approached as a plant. In this model, disease is a mismatch between the inner body and the outer world, and the doctor is most like a gardener, fussing and fiddling, doing a little of this and a little of that. Its way of healing is diffuse, global; it is seeing the patient in the context of his environment, changing what can be changed, and removing what is in the way of the patient's healing on his own. I added that model to my evolving version of medicine.

The version of medicine I saw with my father could not be more different.

In this new model, the body is seen as a computer, or rather as a collection of computers, which are our cells. Disease is an error in the program that runs those cells—our DNA code—and its way of healing is to edit and rewrite that incorrect code. So the doctor is a data provider and programmer, and the patient is a source of data. The body itself is simply an interface, a screen, the outer reflection of an inner code. So its way of healing is at a distance, hands-off; analytic and without a soul—by design.

I don't know how successful this version of medicine will turn out to be. But what I do know is that no matter how useful it is to imagine the body sometimes as a machine, sometimes as a plant, and perhaps also sometimes as a computer, the real body of the patient is none of these. It isn't just more complicated than a machine, plant, or computer—it is Other to anything we can imagine. The only model that could represent it as it really is would be itself.

The Way of Healing associated with that real body is uncanny. It is inductive rather than deductive; interdependent. It is a Way in which there is a give-and-take between body and caregiver, patient and doctor; a mutually constitutive Way among every organ, every cell, and every process. A feel for it developed in me only gradually, over many years of seeing patients, of watching, observing, and practicing. I knew it; I used it; but for a long time I had no way of thinking about it.

And then Slow Food arrived.

"Slow Food"—so counterculture!—so counter to our culture of fast, focus, and fixing or throwing away. Like the body I had come to know, "Slow Food" was subtle and relational, with its emphasis not on the goal but on the process; its insight that the quality of the ingredients and the way of doing something determine the end, that the way *to* something has to be the way *of* it.

Only then did I have a way of thinking about the version of medicine I knew.

It was "Slow Medicine."

I wasn't the only person to come up with this concept. All over the world, many others have independently arrived at the notion of Slow Medicine. Slow Medicine is in the air, and an important model for the future, for all of us to understand.

So what I have done in this book is to collect the moments when some element, some facet, of this Way of Healing revealed itself to me. A doctor holding up his hands—his healing hands—to show me, with a smile. A nurse standing in a doorway, about to go out, get in her car, and save a life. A patient presenting me with the gift of his one-minute-from-fatal aneurism, floating in a glass jar—symbol, as you shall see, of everything that goes to make up Slow. Which is not simply soul but also expertise, knowledge, hard work, logic, and Method.

I have done this because I believe that if you, too, experience what I experienced, you will be brought to the same conclusion about what we need to make our medicine the medicine we deserve. We don't need to remake our health-care system or rebuild it from the ground up. We don't need to do very much. It's pretty simple, quite attainable. Just an added perspective and a change of pace.

It would take me many years and many adventures to discover this Way, however, and I would start to find it even before I started to look. Because I wasn't anyone you would have expected to be wandering on that particular path, nor was it a path I expected myself to wander on. It would start long before I became a doctor, when everything that was going to happen was beginning to pop, the first bubbles appearing on a very particular brew.

The concept hadn't been invented yet, when I got my first taste of Slow.

ONE

On the Cusp of Aquarius

I t started at a particularly unusual time.

All times are unusual, of course, never to be repeated, one of a kind, but this time and place were especially unusual. A revolution was brewing and I was at the center of it, though I didn't know it. Just around the corner from my university was Xerox PARC, where Steve Jobs was being entranced by the mouse and imagining a personal computer. Thirty-five miles to the north was Haight-Ashbury, with its hippies and their counterculture, a revolution of color, scent, sex, and style. Fifty miles to the northeast was Berkeley, where students were occupying parks and making radical demands, and forty miles to the south was Santa Cruz, where the organic food movement was sprouting.

And I was in college, living in a rather strange house that would affect my point of view for the rest of my life.

I'd been in a dormitory until the university, in a first tick of that clock of revolution, rescinded its rule that women live on campus, check into their dormitories before midnight, and see male guests only downstairs. So I began to look around for a different kind of place, and I found it on a bulletin board in the Student Union:

"American family recently returned from Switzerland seeks university student for extra bedroom."

I telephoned and then went over to take a look at the room and meet the family.

The house was just five miles from the university, in the hills where the rich lived in a kind of rural simulacrum, down-to-earth and expensive. I drove down the private lane; in the field on my right, three horses were grazing; in the driveway, chickens were scratching. Jane, the wife, answered the door, and then she showed me around.

The house had been built by a student of Frank Lloyd Wright's, she told me, and it was sprawling, made of adobe and wood, with exposed beams, a heated red concrete floor, and an enormous fireplace with built-in seats. The architect had spared an old oak and built the house around it, so there was a tree growing up through the middle of the living room and out the roof to the sky. Then she took me into the garden, where zucchini and tomatoes were growing in the midst of roses, and then around to the back and I saw the extra bedroom. It had a Swedish slat bed, a sit-down shower, and a teak deck, and looked out onto the Coast Range. It was exotic and peaceful, and I took it.

In that house I would get to be a sort of hippie.

"Sort of" because it was a nice house near the fine university I attended, I was supported by my parents, and I didn't take drugs. "Hippie" because we experimented. The Neumanns had just returned from Switzerland after a twelve-year stay, and their three daughters, though in theory American, spoke English with a Swiss-German accent. They brought back with them the Swiss living they'd learned: washing on Monday, ironing on Tuesday, waxing the floors on Wednesday. Also the six-month supply of food mandated in Switzerland, which were forty-pound tins in the garage, of wheat, rye, and beans.

They also brought back with them a certain worldview. It was what the French call the *longue durée*, and very different from my American worldview. From its perspective, the Romans had only been passing through, and the Middle Ages were not so long ago. The Renaissance, Reformation, and Enlightenment were recent, and America was a charming, puzzling blip on the screen. It was a worldview that tried out each new period, preserved what worked, discarded what didn't, and added what worked to its older ways of being in the world. Many of those ways were remarkably similar to the new ways Americans were discovering, I would learn. Organic food. Meditative spirituality. Political rebelliousness. The congruence of right living, satisfying living, and happy living.

Jane was Mom. She was from an old California family and American through and through. She'd intended to become a biologist, but she married Walter instead and became a wife. In Switzerland she became a perfect wife, obeying the recycling the Swiss did even back then not because of laws but because of their frugal aesthetics. It was wasteful to discard anything usable, she explained to me one day. So every Swiss home had six bins—a white-glass bin, a green-glass bin, a neither-white-nor-green-glass bin, a paper bin, a compost bin, and a trash bin, and the neighbors knew just how much trash was in the trash bin. They also knew whether you washed on Monday, ironed on Tuesday, and waxed on Wednesday.

In Switzerland they'd lived in the village of Kusnacht on Lake Zurich. Carl Jung lived up the street, and Marie-Louise von Franz, Jung's most famous disciple, had herself analyzed Jane. Jane was brilliant but diaphanous; unchallenging, vague, distant. She was like the bird that wandered into the house one day and threw itself against every window trying to get out.

What she brought to the house was a certain Way—perhaps Swiss, perhaps Jung, perhaps her grandparents', perhaps her very own. It was the way we would eventually call Slow and included Indian gurus and the first organic food I ever ate. I would get back from the university and find the newest guru sitting at the table by the oak tree, surrounded by disciples and the smell of curry, incense, floor wax, and laundry. Jane was the Queen, the Moon, a Jungian extroverted feeling type.

Naturally Walter, her husband, was an introverted thinking type. He was tall and thin, and his hair was turning white. His thick mustache was white already. He rode a bicycle to his work as the director of bioengineering at one of the first high-tech companies in Silicon Valley, which focused on electromagnetic equipment. One evening he came home and explained to us how the new technology he was working on would revolutionize agriculture. A Green Revolution would feed the world, he said, because the NMR (MRI) machine they'd invented could analyze the protein content of seeds without damaging them. Jane, the guru, and the disciples listened politely, and then went back to discussing whether the soul could exist apart from the body. Perhaps in reaction Walter became a part-time sandal maker. He would sit at his wooden bench, cut leather, and sew sandals with an awl. With his long, thin legs sticking up as he sat on his bench, he looked like Geppetto, Pinocchio's creator, and in lieu of diaphanous words you had a pair of sandals that lasted until you lost them.

Of the three daughters, Nan was the middle one, and the most fräulein. She had a merry face with flawless skin untouched by sun and nourished by snow. She had straight black hair and observant, very blue eyes. She was tall, healthy, and young, and she gave me my first taste of Slow.

She would get into the tins of wheat, rye, and beans and make up recipes for bread. She might grind the wheat with the rye and then add nuts, cumin, even red pepper. This particular time she did not even use yeast.

I was sitting at the table and watching her as she kneaded the coarse flour with her hands. She worked the dough in a kind of abstraction, then formed it into a loaf and put it in the oven. It didn't rise, of course, without yeast, but its smell filled the kitchen and people began to appear from around the house, drawn by its fragrance.

Finally Nan took the loaf out of the oven. It was small, dense, and primitive, and I'd never seen bread like that. The only bread I knew was Wonder Bread. I watched as she sliced the loaf in the thinnest of slices and then we spread it with the butter she'd also made with the cream Jane had bought from a faraway organic dairy. I had never tasted anything like it. It was gritty, salty, peppery. It took me a long time to chew and had many flavors, and as I tasted, I suddenly understood why, in all the diets I'd ever known, bread was bad for you, and yet the Bible called bread the "staff of life." The Bible didn't mean Wonder Bread but Nan's bread. Perhaps for the dietician, the difference between the two breads is simply in price and nutritional content, but to my palate, they were not even comparable, the difference between them being so obvious, and yet indefinable.

That was my first taste of Slow.

I met Meg, daughter number one, when she decided to come home. She'd run off with her ex-Vietnam-medic boyfriend Peter, but then, several months into my stay, Jane announced that Meg was pregnant and was moving back into my bedroom so she could give birth on the teak deck, or, in bad weather, in bed. Which she did, soon enough.

In the meantime, I was out of a bedroom. But I didn't want to leave. That place was a master's degree in the future. There were the Indian gurus, the organic food, Walter's new technologies. There were the discussions at the dinner table about physics, time, politics; draft resisting, civil disobedience, and government propaganda. There were the marijuana brownies; there was Steve Jobs's little box where you could make phone calls for free; there were the horses, the chickens and our own eggs. We were vegetarians. Walter knew wine. So I did not want to leave.

I looked around for where else I could sleep. I started with the storage room in the horse paddock, but I finally settled on the roof, which, thanks to Frank Lloyd Wright's architect-disciple, was flat. It, too, looked onto the Coast Range and it had large eaves I could move under when it rained, and there I lived until I finished college. It turned out to be a great place to sleep because all night long, I could watch the stars moving across the sky, and I had never seen that before.

Walter taught me the constellations he knew, and one night he explained to me about the "precession of the equinoxes." Because of the wobble of the earth's axis, every year the sky shifts eastward—about 1 degree every 70 years, 30 degrees every 2,000 years, and 360 degrees—one complete revolution—in approximately 26,000 years, which the ancients called the "Great Year." They had measured the precessional shift by whatever zodiacal constellation was appearing on the horizon at the spring equinox. There were twelve such constellations, and each spanned about 30 degrees, a different one appearing every 2,000 years. They believed that whichever constellation that was, characterized the 2,000-year epoch. For us it was Pisces, the Fishes, right above our heads.

Walter pointed it out to me—two not-very-bright stars the ancients envisioned as two fish swimming in opposite directions. The nature of Pisces was therefore, he said, dichotomy, strife, and war—and was what gave our age, the Age of Pisces, its characteristic quality of opposition. Now, however, the constellation of Aquarius was beginning to appear on the horizon, and that would mean a new age, with different strengths and weaknesses.

Often during those nights on the roof, I would wake up and look at the sky, and so I learned for myself how the Big Dipper turns around the North Star like a clock hand, and how the planets wander along the ecliptic. I saw for myself how Venus was some years the morning star in winter and the evening star in spring, and other years the opposite, and during those years I always knew where Mars was, and Saturn, Jupiter, Mercury. I could tell the day of the month by the moon, and the time of night by the stars.

Perhaps that seems of antiquarian interest only, but it was not. Learning that the sky creates a special kind of time—not linear, scientific, progressive time, but seasonal, horticultural, circular time—would be crucial for me later on, when I discovered the Middle Ages and Hildegard of Bingen and their way of understanding the cosmos. Which was circular, not linear, the time of the seasons, which we still wear on our wrists—a revolutionary time, as in the Latin *revolvere*, to turn back, to turn around.

Meg gave birth not on the teak deck but in my ex-bedroom.

On the morning of the birth, she got up and announced that the baby would be born that day. Then she washed my car. Then she went into my ex-room and lay down on the bed and Peter lay down next to her. We gathered around and waited, and then after about two hours, Peter had her start to push. She did, and to my complete surprise, some black thing appeared between her legs, and two pushes later, an entire whole baby, a tiny infant girl, whom Peter did not slap and who did not cry and who breathed very fine without that.

It was stunning. It was like watching a rabbit being pulled out of a hat. There was nothing and then there was something. The tiny thing was covered with a sort of dust, and Jane took her away, cleaned her up, and put her naked next to Meg.

Then the afterbirth came. Meg said she'd heard that some Berkeley vegetarians sautéed and ate it—high in protein and good for your immune system—but we nixed the idea and Peter buried it in the backyard. Then she got up and we had dinner.

Later in medical school I would deliver quite a few babies, with IVs, needles and scissors, fetal scalp monitoring and epidurals. Despite the technology, there was always that same sense of sleight of hand—How did *that* get *here*? Of some amazing magician, who happened in those instances to be me. But there was never that sense of easiness of Meg's birthing, of rolling down a hill—of smoothness, inevitability, slowness.

B<small>Y</small> then I'd finished college and I didn't know what to do next. Most of us didn't, given the times, but especially the women didn't. We had never thought that far ahead. We had seen that all the women we knew were wives and mothers, so presumably some kind of transformation would happen to us in college. But it hadn't happened. I didn't want to have a career as a wife. I didn't want to get a PhD, either, which was the only other option I could think of. So instead I went traveling. That's what we did. It wasn't expensive then—three dollars got you a bed and a breakfast. I bought an open-ended plane ticket, flew to Europe, and spent months adventuring.

And then in an out-of-the-way bookstore I discovered what I would do next.

I hadn't seen a bookstore in a long while and I was delighted. It was dusty and smelled like paper, and in one alcove there was a carousel with books in English. I stood in front of it and spun it and read the spines of the books as it went round. Sinclair Lewis, Herman Wouk, Ernest Hemingway. C. G. Jung, *Memories, Dreams, Reflections.* I pulled that one out. I'd heard of Jung, and Jane had lived in Kusnacht and been analyzed by von Franz, but I'd never read him.

Now, in those days I didn't buy books; they were too expensive. So I stood in front of that carousel all afternoon and simply read through Jung's memoir. What struck me most on that first reading was the quality of his life.

As a student he, too, had been torn between the sciences and the humanities. What he really wanted to be was an archaeologist, but he needed to make a living, and he compromised by becoming a doctor. Then he compromised again by taking an unprestigious but secure job at Zurich's state mental hospital. And then because of that very compromise, his life opened up. He spent years at that hospital, saw his patients every day, listened to them intently, and came to believe that their psychoses weren't always incomprehensible. There were recurring characters in their hallucinations, similar to the characters in fairy tales, myths, and dreams—a young boy, a seductive woman, a villain, a wise old man. There were recurring themes—of adventure, heroism, battle. The patients' hallucinations, Jung began to think, might be understood as stories, with beginnings, middles, and ends.

Then he set up his life so that he could elaborate on his insight. In the mornings he would see patients, and in the afternoons he would study alchemy, astrology, and the traditions of East and West. Eventually he built himself a medieval hideaway, his own private stone house on the shore of Lake Zurich, where there was no electricity and where he alone had the key.

By the end of the afternoon, I did buy the book and read it for a second time, more carefully.

In that second reading I began to see that Jung was explaining things I'd always been aware of but had never had the words for. He was describing the components of the inner world that make up our Self.

There was, for starters, the *shadow*, our own personal shadow—which is everything we reject in ourselves and love to hate in others. Jung called it the "shadow" because it is cast by the light of consciousness, which is why we can't get rid of it. In dreams it appears as a dark figure pursuing the dreamer down a dark path, or sometimes as an animal. It is made up of the parts of yourself that *are* your self but you don't like them. Denying our shadow, projecting it onto others, leaves us frayed and incomplete, he believed, on the alert for the badness of others. Acknowledging our shadow allows us to be whole.

There was the *anima*—the beautiful princess locked in the castle whom we so want to rescue—which is also a part of ourselves and the woman we seek in women. There was the corresponding *animus*—the handsome hero we want to marry or become, or both.

And there was the intriguing implication of a kind of recursiveness to these particular opposites. Since every woman has an *animus*, a male image or male part of her Self, that inner image must also have *its own anima*; and every man's *anima* its own *animus*. So a woman would have not only an ideal image of a man within her, but also a secondary image of the kind of woman that inner man would want. A man's internal female image, his *anima*, would have her own reflected secondary male image, the *animus* of his *anima*, and which one would he decide to be?

And underneath all, as a kind of ocean or soft bottom of a lake, was the most important character of all, the unconscious, the *Unbewusste*—the behind-the-scenes observer that thinks in pictures and has its own plan. It gives us hints of its plan in our dreams, in accidents, in serendipity, Jung wrote. Its purpose is "individuation," the powerful, un-Darwinian urge to become our Self, to unite all these disparate characters, feelings, and perspectives into a whole, but a whole whose wholeness we can never see.

There was even more, I realized, as I read the book for a third time. Jung had a philosophy of the wholeness of things. Everything implies its opposite and nothing is true unless its opposite is also true. Evil and good, night and day, dark and light, are all of a piece, and to be "whole" means not rejecting but experiencing the Other. Jung didn't believe in progress but he did believe in development. The motive force for change was *enantiodromia*, the confrontation of the opposites, the giving birth to the opposite by means of confrontation. He believed in circularity, in turning, rotation—that cyclical time I'd observed on the Neumanns' roof. Later I would find out that his was a very old theory, a turning based on the precession of the equinoxes, a return, and a completion of a Great Year.

It was Jung who first called the coming new age the "Age of Aquarius." As the dawn equinoctial sky slips from Pisces into Aquarius, he wrote, we will experience new ways of looking at things, ways we once knew but during the Age of Pisces were pushed underground, into the dark muck of the unconscious. The Age of Aquarius will be a revolution, he wrote, and we were just on the cusp.

After I finished the book for the third time, I knew it was what I wanted. That infusing of past into present, especially of the West's premodern sensibility, cut off by modernity.

But how?

I would become a Jungian analyst, that's what I would do.

I've always thought it serendipity that brought me to that out-of-the-way bookstore with *Memories, Dreams, Reflections* in its carousel. Jung would have called it synchronicity—his concept for explaining meaningful events that have no Newtonian cause. The accidental meeting that changes a life, the prophetic dream, the accurate intuition. He connected synchronicity to the ancient idea of the "sympathy of all things," which was why every morning he greeted his pots and pans with "Good morning, Pot, good morning, Pan," and which is why, when people get cancer, they take it personally.

So as soon as I got back home from my travels, I contacted the Jung Institute to find out how to become a Jungian analyst. I would need a doctorate first, they told me—in psychology or medicine.

That was fine with me. After six months in the real world, I was ready for the longest possible stay away and I chose medicine.

TWO

Dr. Gurushantih and My New White Coat

For the first two years, medical school was just like the school I'd been used to. There were classrooms, professors, and homework. And yet there were differences; there was a different tone and a different goal and a different kind of knowledge. The tone was set by the professors, who were not like the professors I'd had in college, pursuing knowledge for its own sake. Their PhDs were not in the humanities but in anatomy, physiology, and microbiology, and their interests were in experimenting on animals, tissues, and cells. As professors in a medical school, however, their job was to make sure we knew what medical doctors were supposed to know about their specialties, which were the facts.

Unconnected facts, as it turned out, brought to light by all their different experiments—some on the frog, some on bacteria, some on cells in a petri dish. And unlike in mathematics or physics, their facts did not all fit together. There was no structure on which to hang them and we just had to memorize them. Frog kidney chemistry, rat pressure-resistance equations, bacterial enzyme cascades, intermittent accidental glimpses of the elephants' skin or trunk or toe, and we were the blind men, trying to figure out what that thing—the human body—actually was.

At the same time—and this was also different from college—each one of those facts was important. Each one might mean life or death, depending on whether we remembered or forgot it. If we forgot that patients with severe lung disease lost their carbon dioxide drive and we gave them too much oxygen, they could stop breathing. If we forgot a certain drug interaction and gave our patient an incompatible drug, he could die. There were thousands of such life-saving but disconnected facts to memorize, and medical school was stressful in a way that regular school had never been.

But into the bargain, I was a female medical student.

It had been 128 years since Elizabeth Blackwell graduated from medical school, the first woman to do so since the creation of medical schools in twelfth-century Paris. Yet of our school's 120 professors, only two were female. In the entire school, there were only seventeen women: the sophomore class had four; the junior class, three; and the senior class, one. My class was the first year for which there'd been a concerted effort not to reject women. So there were nine of us in a class of seventy-seven.

The eight women ahead of us did try to help us out. On the first weekend of our first year, they gave us a potluck and some tips. Try not to let the men crowd you out on rounds. Watch out for Dr. Smith's hands. If all else fails and you're about to be asked yet another obscure question you don't have the answer to, stare at their trousers.

On the Monday after the potluck, Dr. Leuger, Head of Anatomy, and rumored to be an ex-Nazi, stationed himself at the door of the anatomy classroom. He was slim and straight with cropped white hair and pale blue eyes, and as we squeezed past him, he murmured to each of us:

"I hear zat ze vimmen are organ-eye-zink."

I'd never before felt like a female student. But there were the dirty jokes at the beginning of the lectures to wake us up, the *Playboy* slides in the middle to keep us awake, and a disconcerting professorial attention to our long hair and feminine faces.

And the students were different from the students I was used to. By "students" I mean the male students. They had clear goals—finish medical school, get a good residency, make a nice living—and yet they had no edge. They were nice, soft, and agreeable. If something didn't make sense, they did not object. Although neither did we women. We were all adrift. It was as if we were a few turns into a maze. We couldn't see over the sides, we couldn't turn around, we could only put one foot in front of us and hope for the best.

At the same time, we all felt—something. Something was going on. There were draft-card burnings, Black Panthers, Christopher Street. There were struggles for abortion, birth control, patients' rights, alternative medicine. Acupuncture and Chinese medicine arrived. Farmers' markets. All starting right then. There was a stirring, a stretching, a waking up.

A Jungian *enantiodromia*—the confrontation of opposites—was preparing, of black/white, men/women, straight/gay, fast/slow—when what is rejected becomes what is accepted, the below turns into the above, and the hidden into the seen. Jung took from Heraclitus the general idea that all things change into their opposites—black into white, femaleness into maleness, yang into yin—because everything has a piece of its opposite within. The *enantiodromia* begins when that first sense of the opposite inside makes its presence known, and it began for me the day I drove into the City to buy my white coat.

I already had a white coat, but it was the wrong white coat. I'd had to buy it for the first day of medical school. It was a long lab coat and I was proud of it until the end of that second year, when I realized that the third-year medical students didn't wear long white coats. They wore short white jackets and, wearing them, they, that is, the men students, looked like real doctors. So now we all wanted a short white jacket, and finally, for the physical diagnosis course at the end of those first two years, we were told to buy one.

Later we would discover that the interns—the medical students who'd finished medical school but were now earning their license in a first year of real doctoring—never wore short white jackets. What was cool for them, who were so confident, so busy, was not to wear a white coat at all, but to drape their stethoscopes around their necks. They didn't need the big pockets in the white jacket, not for the *Washington Manual*—they had all its wisdom in their heads—not for equipment—they just grabbed whatever was around—not for the index cards of their patients, which they kept in their back pocket. That's when we would get rid of our short white jackets. Until, six years later, at the end of my training, I would see that the real doctors, the attendings, wore . . . long white lab coats, which provided the best protection for their clothes.

The white coats, that is to say, were symbol and proof that medicine was a guild, with a strict hierarchy, with steps up the stairway that you took not when you felt you were ready but when you were permitted. First-year medical student. Third-year medical student. Intern. Resident. Attending. You had to learn what was necessary, as decided by those who went before you, those who knew. You had to go up the steps, learn in order, no skipping, slow.

There's something to be said for that kind of structure.

There were no uniform stores near the medical school, but my friend and fellow medical student, Rosalind, knew where I could find one, so I drove up to the specialized uniform store she told me about. I spent some time looking through its racks, searching for that short white jacket. I found nurses' coats in pink polyester and woman-sized lab-tech coats with cinched waists and tiny pockets, but no short doctor jackets in my size. Finally the saleslady explained: There were no doctor's coats for women. There were only men's and the smallest was size 28. She showed it to me. It was heavy cotton with two enormous pockets for a stethoscope and medical manual, but the pièce de résistance were its hidden slits for putting your hands in your trouser pockets without taking off your jacket. So that's what I bought.

And then I went exploring. I'd heard that there was a women's bookstore in the area and I wanted to see it. It was only a few blocks from the uniform shop without doctors' coats for women.

This is where the *enantiodromia* began for me, the confrontation between the opposites represented by the term "woman doctor." It was a syllogism that couldn't make sense. Doctors were men; women were nurses, and what, then, was a "woman doctor"? One hundred years before, Dr. William Osler, dean of American medicine, had provided one answer: "There are three sexes," he wrote, "men, women, and women doctors."

There wasn't much to go on. Neither feminine nor masculine fit the bill. And neutral—neither—didn't either.

The overlarge man's white coat was helpful, but only in a limited way. It answered the question: how did I want to appear, how did I want to be treated? But it didn't solve it completely. *Persona* was Jung's word for how we appear to others. He took it from the Latin word for mask—*persona*—in ancient theater, actors wore masks that had a hole, the *persona*, for the voice to come through. Your *persona* tells the world at first glance who you are; how to treat you; what you see yourself as; what you should be taken for. Before medical school it had been simple: my *persona* was girl, woman, student. But now that I was about to be in the hospital as a medical student, as a pre-doctor, how was I to appear? *Persona* was made manifest by clothes and style, voice and gesture, talk and silence, gait and stride—how to be a woman in a man's profession?

The syllogism was: Doctors make decisions, which means, in the end, sometimes saying no; that was what, in part, we would be learning. Women, on the other hand, smile and always say yes, even if they mean no. Women who do say no, who push back, who make a decision and carry it out regardless, are, depending on the century, viragos, bluestock-ings, castrators (Freud), *animus*-possessed (Jung), or feminists. So how was I to be that contradiction in terms, that third sex—a woman doctor?

The bookstore was on the main street, almost hidden between two buildings. When I walked in, a little bell jingled. There was a large woman behind the counter in the corner, with a big face and very short hair. Otherwise, all there was in that bookstore were books. By women. Everywhere. I had no idea we'd written so much. On shelves lining the walls, in bookcases that filled the space like a library. Fiction, history, psychology, spirituality, politics.

I bought three: Simone de Beauvoir's *Second Sex*, Radclyffe Hall's *Well of Loneliness*, and a journal with the shocking name *Amazon Quarterly*—revolutionary works as much as, or even more than, Marx. Then I drove back to medical school.

The physical diagnosis course was where we'd see real patients for the first time, and it came at the end of those first two years. There were three other students in my section, and we drove over together to meet our preceptor, Dr. Gurushantih.

He was at the VA Hospital, which was seven floors high, rising from a sea of asphalt, and looked more like an office building than a hospital. Inside there were pale green walls, linoleum floors, and aluminum win-dows, and we took the elevator to the fourth floor. Dr. Gurushantih met us. He was young, handsome, and enthusiastic, and in a lilting Indian-English accent explained that what we would do that afternoon would be walk around and see the patients he'd picked out for us. He would explain to us their diagnoses and then show us how we could arrive at the diagnosis just by examining the patient.

He was a pulmonologist, a lung specialist, he told us, and the first patient he showed us had the fingernails you get when you have chronic pulmonary disease. He lifted up the patient's hand and demonstrated the nails. They were curved and splayed and gray, not pink. See how the angle where the nail bed comes out of the tip of the finger is gone? That is called "clubbing" and is diagnostic of chronic pulmonary disease. We could count on it.

I looked at my own nails. I had never noticed before. There was a crisp angle where the base of the nail came out of the tip of my finger.

We walked over to the next patient. He had a pleural effusion, Dr. Gurushantih said. This is liquid that is inside the chest but outside the lungs, and can accumulate if there is lung cancer or a lung infection or heart failure, but he didn't know yet which it was. So what he was going to do now was drain the fluid with a needle and then send it to the lab for diagnosis.

We gathered around as Dr. Gurushantih explained the procedure to the patient and then sat on the bed. His warm brown hands tapped the patient's back from top to bottom and we listened carefully. We could hear the sound his tapping made go from hollow to thud, and where it changed timbre was the level of the fluid. Dr. G took his pen out of his white coat pocket and made a mark where we heard the change. He felt for the rib below the pen mark, numbed the area, and then with total confidence stuck a long needle into the chest.

Fluid began to drip from it. We watched as he attached a connector to a vacuum bottle, which filled up with clear yellow fluid. That was a good sign, he told us; its yellow clarity meant the patient probably didn't have cancer or an infection but heart failure, and that would be easy to treat. During the whole time, the patient hadn't said anything, but when Dr. G said it wasn't cancer, we could see his shoulders drop and he took a deep breath. Then Dr. G took the needle out, put a Band-Aid over the site, and we went to the next patient.

This patient had a brain tumor. And since the skull is a bone box, it can't distend as a tumor enlarges, so as the tumor grows, it puts pressure on everything inside the box—the soft brain, the fluid that cushions the brain, and the cable of nerves that goes from brain to the retina of the eye. Naturally that cable, called the optic nerve, swells from the pressure, and you can see that swelling if you look at the retina with your ophthalmoscope.

We all took out our ophthalmoscopes and looked, and I could see it! The optic nerve was a yellowish disc at the back of the eye, and because of the pressure that the brain tumor was exerting, its edges were not sharp and crisp but blurry. This, Dr. G said, meant that he had "hydrocephalus," a swelling of the brain, and it was how we could diagnose increased intracranial pressure.

We didn't even know how to take a blood pressure, and he showed us that, too; the four measurements you can get and what each means for diagnosis.

All afternoon we followed Dr. G around, and he introduced us to patients who let every one of us look at their fingernails, tap their chests, and squint into our ophthalmoscopes. It was an eye-opener, a brain-opener, and a heart-opener. If I examined patients, I learned that day, I could diagnose disease. Brain tumors, lung infections, heart disease. It was so interesting, so powerful, that slow, thoughtful, and methodical exam.

I was inspired.

So I went out and bought a copy of the book Dr. G recommended, *Bedside Diagnostic Examination*, by Elmer L. DeGowin and Richard L. DeGowin, known simply as DeGowin and DeGowin. It was the bible of the physical exam, he explained, and it looked like a Bible. It had a soft brown cover, 560 tissue-thin pages, and it described every sign of disease that could be found on the physical exam. There were thousands of such signs, and, unlike all those disconnected facts we'd spent the first two years learning, DeGowin and DeGowin's facts had a structure: they followed the body, from head to toe. So all the physical signs of the scalp, skull, eyes, ears, nose, and throat were written there, all the way down to the toenails. I outlined it and made index cards of it, and put them in my white jacket's breast pocket.

Then, on the last day of the course, Dr. G gave each of us a patient to completely examine. We were to see how much we could glean about him and his diagnoses simply by examining his body.

My patient was Mr. Alan Pointer, fifty-six years old. He had a gravelly voice, big ears, a crew cut, and a tattoo of an anchor on his right shoulder, so he was a classic VA patient, though I didn't know that yet. I introduced myself, pulled the curtain around his bed, and began going through my index cards. I asked him every question, and did every test, from head to toe. It took me four hours, and by the time I was done we were both sweating and exhausted. It was evening and Dr. G came looking for me, and I had the sense that I had overdone it, just a bit.

But I appreciate Mr. Pointer to this day. Because doing that one full and complete DeGowin and DeGowin exam was amazing. It was like making pottery or woodworking—detailed, precise, careful. It was my first inkling that medicine was not only a science but also a craft. Everything mattered, everything was important and told a story. The patient's hands—their warmth and dryness or cold and wetness; their nails, palms, pulse; the texture of their skin and hair; the presence or absence of lymph nodes—and that was just up to the elbow.

That day, Dr. G convinced me that if I examined a patient completely, I could tell what he did and didn't have. Not everything he did or didn't have, but a lot of it. And that if I did *not* do a thorough exam, there was no good way to tell, even with all the technology in the world. The patient's body was a continent to map, and you talk about discovery! Why would I ever want to be an armchair explorer? It was the very first piece, and perhaps the most important piece, of what I would end up calling Slow Medicine. When all else fails, examine the patient.

I would never forget what Dr. G taught me. I would mentally thank him many times, when the examination of the patient's scalp revealed unexpected metastatic esophageal cancer as the reason for his weakness, or when examination of the fingers showed the rare disease of pseudo-pseudohypoparathyroidism. That exam was the rock, the foundation of Medicine. After all, what is it the patient brings us? Even if it's his suffering mind, it is most often expressed in his suffering body.

The next thing I would be convinced of would be method, the power of the methodical going-through of a patient's record page by page, the learning of the story, which would be precisely what would be left out of my father's care—or really, not left out but rendered impossible by technology.

THREE

The Man with a
Hole in His Head

Since I was planning to be a Jungian analyst, my first clerkship would be psychiatry, which included neurology because medicine was not certain about which came first, the mind or the brain.

On the one hand, from its work on hysteria in the nineteenth century, psychiatry knew that mind affects brain and could cause physical symptoms such as headaches, blindness, or even paralysis. On the other hand, neurology knew from its work with pathology and the microscope that brain could affect mind. Meningitis, encephalitis, strokes, and cancers all could cause psychoses and confusion. So psychiatry and neurology went together, and in the clerkship we learned them both.

But they were very different. On Psychiatry we hardly ever examined our patients' brains or bodies. We were supposed to and we did try, but a confused, agitated, or psychotic patient rarely permitted a physical exam. On Neurology, though, the physical examination was key. It even had its own neurologic exam, separate from the physical exam Dr. Gurushantih had taught us, and it was the main thing we were to learn during our month on the neurology ward, which was also at the VA Hospital.

On our first day, the resident, Craig, took us on a tour of his patients and demonstrated that special exam to us. There were eight parts of it, he explained, starting with examining the head and neck, then the cranial nerves, the reflexes, strength, sensation, gait, and balance. And there were special tools, developed mostly in the nineteenth century when neurology came into its own, for each part of the exam. We watched as he took them one by one out of his scuffed black bag. A flashlight. A hammer. A pin, a tuning fork, a stick, the key to your mistress's house.

We balked at the key. Really?

Well, that was what the discoverer of the test, Monsieur le docteur Babinski, had used, what he taught his own students to use, and what Craig himself used—the key to his mistress's, actually his girlfriend's, house. The key was for testing the Babinski reflex on the sole of the foot, which was an excellent test for dementia, he told us. When you're born, the sole of your foot splays upward and outward when stroked, but as the brain develops, the sole learns to curl inward and downward. In dementia, which some call the second childhood, that infant reflex, the Babinski reflex, returns. The sole splays outward when it is stroked with a key. He supposed we could use some other key, but, hey, there was tradition to think of.

The most exotic thing Craig had in his black bag was a box of scents for testing cranial nerve number one, the olfactory nerve. They were little glass bottles with steel caps and contained essential oils of rosemary, violet, lavender, and cedar. I saw only one other neurologist ever test cranial nerve number one, and Craig having that box in his bag, and using it, was a measure for me—and still is—of his devotion to his craft. The neurologic exam he taught was a beautiful exam. A careful neurologist can often make the diagnosis from it alone. Even today, neurologists have not yet given up their beautiful exam, although I expect they will shortly.

But it was the physical finding he showed us on Corporal Eks that impressed me the most.

Corporal Eks was a handsome young black guy, sitting up in bed, dressed. There were no IVs or oxygen around his bed, and it wasn't obvious that he had any kind of medical problem, except that his skull had been shaved and his hair was beginning to grow in. He seemed pretty chipper as he answered Craig's questions about where he was and how he was feeling. He was bright and alert and his answers seemed correct.

Then Craig asked us, why did we think Corporal Eks was here? What did we think he had?

He must have had brain surgery a while ago, was the best we could do.

"Why don't you palpate his skull?" Craig instructed us, with a gleam in his eye.

Now, palpating the skull is a part of the physical exam, but hardly anyone ever does it. It's not complicated. You put your hands on the patient's head and feel the hair, its quality and thickness, the scalp, for rashes and lesions, and then the skull for lumps and bumps. Perhaps it's a remnant of the nineteenth-century science of phrenology, when the bumps on the skull were thought to be diagnostic of disease.

Corporal Eks's skull looked perfectly fine. Since it was shaved, you could see it well. So we looked over to Craig. Why bother to palpate it?

By way of answer he put his fingers on the top of Corporal Eks's head and pressed, and his fingers went all the way down. Then he let go, and the dent bounced back, like he'd been pressing on a balloon filled with water. He explained. Even though Corporal Eks looked fine, spoke fine, answered fine, and his skull appeared to be intact—it wasn't and he wasn't. Five months before, he'd fractured his skull and then sustained a subdural hematoma that became infected. The neurosurgeons had to remove a large piece of his skull on the right and much of the infected brain underneath. Corporal Eks could still listen, answer, and talk because the right side of the brain in a right-handed person is, to some extent, extra.

After that I never left out of my physical exam a careful palpation of the skull.

Unlike the other clerkships I would have later, in neurology I had no responsibility for patients. My job was to learn the neurologic exam by practicing on Craig's patients, and then afterward to read about their diagnoses.

So I spent quite a bit of time in Craig's office, which was a windowless room on the ward with a desk and chairs, curling yellowed schedules on the walls, and charts piled on floor and desk. Toward the end of the month we were sitting in it together when Craig began telling me about Patient Harris, who had just been readmitted.

Mr. Harris was sixty-two and had been a successful lawyer, Craig told me, wealthy, respected, buffered. Then about five years ago, unexpectedly, his wife died and he became first depressed, then very depressed, then suicidally depressed, and then manic. He decided all of a sudden to sell his house, and did so for considerably less than it was worth. Then he took the money and invested it in various manic schemes. He lost it all, of course, and slowly descended the social register, ratchet by ratchet.

By this time I understood that mania was depression's other face. Some people can get only so depressed before they switch all at once from negative to positive, from depressed to manic.

Mr. Harris became high, excited, and cheerful to the max, Craig recounted. His law practice fell to pieces, and he was in and out of the psychiatry unit, taking lithium, stopping lithium, pursuing court cases of his own, incorrigible.

Well then, why was he on Neurology? I wanted to know.

"Headaches. Terrible headaches. He's had them for years, and has been admitted to us many times. But we never find anything, and here he is back for yet another workup. He never lets us examine him, though. He throws us out of the room. I don't know why we bother. But—maybe he'll let you examine him. You're new; he's never seen you before. Why don't you go take a look?"

I was still shy—most medical students are, since medical school selects for introverts. But I took my courage, got up, and walked over to his room, which was kitty-corner to our cubbyhole. It was a single room and the door was closed. I knocked and walked in.

Mr. Harris was alone, sitting on the bed, dressed in a short-sleeve white shirt and threadbare slacks, with a battered, ex-nice briefcase on the bed with him. It was open and he was looking through a sheaf of papers in it, which were also battered.

I was a medical student, I told him, and I was learning the neurologic exam. Would he let me examine him?

He looked up from his papers. His black lawyerly glasses were slightly askew. His hair was thinning and uncombed, there was gray stubble on his cheeks, and yet he was still almost handsome. There was a certain elegance about him.

No, he wouldn't. He'd been examined too many times already. His head hurt him terribly and no one ever had an answer. He was tired of it but would I care to go over the papers related to his court cases? He was suing the executor of his wife's estate and also the cleaners who'd ruined his suit. Plus he was trying to get his house back. Someone had forged his signature to the deed, sold it, and disappeared with all the money.

He was moving just a little too fast for me, just a little too jerky, too intense.

"No, no, thanks—maybe some other time," I said, backing out of the room and leaving him reading and turning over his worn papers. I went back to Craig.

"He won't let me examine him."

"No surprise. No one's been able to examine him for years. Why don't you just sit down and go over his chart?"

He pointed to the stack by the desk. "Five years' worth."

On the floor I saw charts piled up to the desktop, and each was as thick as a telephone book. I arranged them chronologically, took the first one, the earliest, off the top, and sat down on a chair in the corner.

I'd never gone through a patient's records before, and Mr. Harris's took me all afternoon.

Going through them, page by page, volume by volume, was much more interesting than I ever would have imagined. What struck me most was how Mr. Harris's chart was a collective enterprise of investigating, documenting, and hypothesizing, and that it was ongoing. It was like a book, with a beginning and a middle, but unlike a book, its authors were writing without knowing the end. What's more, as they were writing their notes, they did not know what might happen next: whether Mr. Harris would die, get well, or get sicker. So I could see the medical thought process at work in the midst of uncertainty, how it made its guesses, its best guesses, and what it did when those guesses didn't pan out.

Also, since the records were all written by hand, I was able to see how the chart was an individual as well as a communal process. I could correlate different scripts with different doctors, nurses, and social workers, both as a group—the surgeons' scrawl, the internists' print, the nurses' convent script—and as individuals. The scripts were characters in the story as well.

Mr. Harris's chart was especially interesting because it included not only his medical admissions but his psychiatric admissions. Later, that would be unusual. A law would be passed by mental health advocates that required a separate set of charts for psychiatric records that only psychiatry could see. But with Mr. Harris I could read the whole thing, psychiatry and neurology together, without splitting off mind from brain.

It did take me all afternoon.

In the first volume I read about his first admission to psychiatry, five years before, when he came in suicidally depressed. I read what the psychiatrist thought, what Mr. Harris told him, and what the nurses and social workers did. I could see the results of his brain tests and his mind tests.

In volume two his mania began, and I could see the medications that were tried and failed, the blood tests, the different medical considerations, and the results of X-rays and consultations.

In volume three, so about three years before, his headaches started, and he had his first admission to neurology. Tests weren't as sophisticated back then. Walter's NMR had not yet turned into the MRI, and CT scans had just been invented. All we had to look inside the brain was the "brain scan" and the ghastly pneumoencephalogram, spinal taps, and blood tests. Mr. Harris had had just about every test that neurology and psychiatry had to offer. Many times. Without a diagnosis, except for "crazy," which wasn't satisfying, and "headache" without any effective treatment.

And then, two-thirds of my way through volume four, so about two years before, there was an intriguing note. Mr. Harris had a high calcium level, and the neurology resident suggested that perhaps he had multiple myeloma, a blood cell cancer that can cause a high calcium and depression and head pain. The resident had recommended a follow-up calcium test to verify the result and a skull X-ray to rule out that possibility.

I looked through volumes four and five to find out what the repeat calcium level had been and what the skull X-ray showed. But Mr. Harris had demanded discharge before those tests were done, and in all the rest of his admissions, the doctors had been dealing with his mania. No one in volume four or five had ever done another calcium test or gotten a skull X-ray.

I didn't know much about multiple myeloma. When we'd learned about it in pathology, it had seemed rare, abstruse. So now, since I had the time, I went over to the hospital library and read up on it. Multiple myeloma was a cancer of plasma cells, I learned, that nested in bone and sometimes produced a chemical that chewed up the bone, causing pain and also an elevated calcium level, as the calcium leached out of the bone into the blood. That high calcium could then cause mental problems—anxiety, agitation, paranoia, and depression. Sometimes the cancer cells also produced a protein that clogged the blood vessels and could cause confusion. Multiple myeloma could smolder for years without manifesting itself.

So when Craig returned to his office in the late afternoon, I asked him, "What about multiple myeloma? Two years ago Mr. Harris had a high calcium and the neurology resident suggested that multiple myeloma with hypercalcemia might explain his symptoms—including his head pain. He was supposed to have had a repeat calcium and a skull film but never did."

That was a pretty interesting idea, Craig said.

He explained our thinking to Mr. Harris, and Mr. Harris agreed to have his skull X-rayed the next day.

Craig and I went downstairs to see the films.

What they showed was classic for multiple myeloma, he told me, and even I could see. Mr. Harris had holes in his head. Little round holes all over his skull. That was why he had terrible head pain, and perhaps also why he had depression, mania, confusion. He would still have to have a bone biopsy for diagnosis, and blood and urine tests, but multiple myeloma, Craig said, was what he almost certainly had. And it would be treatable, he said, and with treatment Mr. Harris's headaches might improve, perhaps even disappear. Who knows, maybe when his calcium came down to normal, his mania, depression, paranoia, and confusion would improve as well. It wasn't curable; he would probably die of the disease eventually, but in the meantime, which could be many years, he would feel better.

It was my very first diagnosis, and I couldn't quite believe it. I was just a medical student—what did I know?

And I hadn't known, either. I had merely seen—*noticed*—in those five thick charts, a single sentence, which was not even my own insight but someone else's: "Perhaps the patient has multiple myeloma." I knew just enough to notice, which was reassuring, because that meant I didn't have to know everything but only enough to recognize that something might be worth pursuing.

Mr. Harris was glad to hear about his diagnosis, although he still would not let me palpate his skull. He did let us get another calcium test, however, which was high, and he did agree to treatment. And he was relieved that a reason had been found for his headaches and that something finally could be done about them.

He didn't give up his court cases, though. Still, it's always better to know, if you have pain, that you are not imagining it; that it is not "in your head" but in your skull; that it is real pain, and that you are believed and taken seriously.

What a lesson that was in Slow-Medicine-to-be! It took me all afternoon, five telephone-book-size charts, page by page. And how important those pages were, to be able to read them, turn them, and go on to the next. Later, when electronic charts replaced those paper pages, such a review would become impossible. Those pages, those charts, embodied story, and with Mr. Harris they proved to me for the first but not the last time the efficiency of what seems, at first glance, to be inefficient.

It would be in the medicine clerkship that I would learn this explicitly from Dr. Greg. He would be my first Slow Medicine doctor, although he wouldn't have known what I mean by that. He would have said that what he practiced and preached was simply—Good Medicine.

FOUR

Dr. Greg's
30 Percent Solution

The County Hospital was at the corner of freeway and mall. It didn't look like much—a plain 1960s utilitarian box of five stories and aluminum windows. Looking at it from the mall, you never would have guessed that inside that building was everything society didn't want to look at or see.

Whenever I walked into it, I was surprised anew by how what was inside it was never outside it. That was, I decided, one of the unsung advantages of our medical system, one of the perks that makes its expense worthwhile even from a businessman's point of view. Ancient Rome had no such system as the county system for taking care of its sick poor, and imagine how bad for business that must have been! The leprotic, the cancerous, the tubercular sitting on the Forum steps, right in the face of the politicians and bargaining businessmen. What a brilliant innovation of the Middle Ages to have had a place—the almshouse, the *hôtel-Dieu*, God's Hotel—where anyone—the sick, the old, the poor—could go and be welcomed inside. All those reminders of our inevitable suffering and mortality tucked away, out of sight, out of mind. Although the mall was just across the street from the hospital, I never, ever, saw a single patient—balding, with IV attached, coughing up blood, gangrenous leg smelling and hanging useless at his side—sitting, lying, or standing in that mall.

But once you entered the hospital, there everything was—sickness, suffering, and death—although you realized this only gradually. The first floor still had a businesslike atmosphere, with offices, executives, carpets, and cafeteria—healthy people mainly, except for the emergency room. And even the emergency room was more mall-like than not. Take a number, hand over your credit card, wait. Only when you stepped into the elevator, pressed the button, and began to ascend did health get out and illness get in.

Second floor—Obstetrics and Pediatrics. Not too bad: birth, new life, happiness, and expectation, and even the sick were young, playful, and relatively attractive.

Third floor—Surgery. Illness was still fixable, there was still hope, no matter how terrible things appeared.

Fourth floor—Neurology. Things began to get dicey.

But it was only on the fifth and last floor, nearest to heaven, when you got to Medicine, that the real challenge to your beliefs and desires would greet you. And Medicine was where I was headed, next.

Death itself—Pathology and the morgue—was down in the basement, trundled below in a special gurney contrived to appear empty of anything as challenging as a corpse.

Medicine would be formative. It would prove to be the Haydn of the specialties, nonchalant in its expertise, its detached cheer, its brilliant method. And it was not only at the top of the hospital but also, at the time, at the top of the medical hierarchy.

It was the gentleman's specialty, untouched by the blood and guts of surgery. The distinction went all the way back to Greece, when

surgeons were low-class craftsmen who worked with their hands—
cheires in Greek—while physicians worked with *physis*—with Nature.
When universities were established in the Middle Ages, that distinction
became even clearer: physicians went to the university and became
"doctors"—from the Latin *doctus*, learned, educated—while surgery
remained a handcraft of drawing blood, pulling teeth, and removing
bladder stones. And although in the nineteenth century, medicine and
surgery did combine, and a medical license today is for medicine *and*
surgery, the two are still, as they have always been, two professions
with different methods, styles, and worldviews.

The medical internist was elegant to watch. Presented with a
complicated case, he would listen intently. He would ask a question or
two, and then go over to the patient and elicit the one piece of information the student had missed, so obtaining the real story that made the
history, physical exam, and lab results fall into place. Then, with soap-
smelling, uncallused hands, he would perform the essential test that
proved his diagnosis, and last, with the 2,600 pages of *Harrison's Principles of Internal Medicine* in memory, defend his conclusion. The
specialty of internal medicine has since fallen down the hierarchy, but at
the time, it was the most prestigious of all.

For medical students it was also the hardest, because we had to stay
in the hospital through the night, because we had to work up patients
on our own, and because we had to draw blood.

Drawing blood was my first problem.

We'd been taught how to draw blood a few months before. When we
were told to pair up, I paired up with my friend Rosalind because before
medical school she'd been a lab tech and already knew how to draw
blood. Syringes, needles, alcohol swabs, and tourniquets were distrib-
uted, and Rosalind said she would teach me by demonstrating on me.

I sat down on a stool and watched. She cleaned my skin with alcohol,
and then she attached the needle to the syringe, put a tourniquet around
my arm, and pushed the needle into the big vein at my elbow. She drew

back the syringe and it filled with blood. She took off the tourniquet, took out the needle, and bandaged the puncture site. Then she filled the test tube with blood and disposed of her equipment. QED.

"Okay, Victoria, now you draw my blood."

She sat on the stool and put out her arm, and I followed her example. Cleanse skin, prepare syringe, put tourniquet around arm, insert needle, withdraw blood, remove needle.

Blood spurted all over the place.

"Take the tourniquet off the arm *before* you remove the needle."

Ah, yes, that's right. Remove tourniquet—*then* withdraw needle, fill tube, dispose of equipment.

I began to feel lightheaded.

"Victoria, you look awful."

The next thing I knew I was waking up and I was on the floor. I'd passed out.

Clearly I would need further instruction before attempting venipuncture on a real patient. So I found Celsa, the lab tech who drew all the morning bloods for the hospital, and asked her to teach me her method. It would turn out to be my first experience of Slow in medicine.

Celsa began by showing me her cart, which was neat and well organized. Here, lined up by size, were the test tubes, and here were the needles, syringes, alcohol swabs, and tourniquets. Keeping everything in order and organized was important, she told me. Then we walked over to her next patient.

Before you do anything, gather all the equipment you'll need.

She did so.

Make sure you have everything, and then arrange it in order on the bedside table: tourniquet, syringe, the proper-size needle, swabs, test tubes, forms.

She did so.

Next—get comfortable. This is important, Celsa emphasized. It might seem more efficient just to walk from bed to bed, tourniquet, puncture, and move on, but don't do that. Because now and again it won't be easy to get blood from someone—drug abusers' arms, the oft-punctured arms of the chronically ill—and if you bend over awkwardly you'll miss the one vein and it will take a long time to find another. You should always sit down to draw blood, Celsa said, on a chair or on the patient's bed. Settle down. Compose yourself.

She showed me what she did on the next patient, and then had me show her. This was the famous medical dictum, "See one, Do one, Teach one," although I didn't know that at the time.

Celsa watched as I sat down and put the tourniquet on the patient's arm, and it was easy. I found the vein, filled the syringe, took the tourniquet off, and did not pass out. And from then on, I always followed her method. Whenever I had to draw blood, I would sit down on the patient's bed and make myself comfortable. I would look at the patient, and sometimes we would even smile at each other. It would take more time but I never forgot to take off the tourniquet, and I rarely missed a vein. Plus, Celsa had given me an added lesson. I had learned that I could sit on the patient's bed, and that sitting created an intimacy, a sharing, a common goal. That getting comfortable, that composing of myself, made a pool of calmness for me and my patient within the crazy cacophony of the hospital. It was my first experience of feeling Slow, of the space and quality of time that Slow creates.

As a medical student I didn't have a necessary task. I was supernumerary. My job was to learn what I could. So when a patient was admitted, first the resident and then the intern would examine him, write the workup and the orders. Then I would go in and redo everything as an exercise. This exhausted the patient, of course, but it was the quid pro quo that the free care of the County Hospital exacted.

Then, after our exam, we, the medical students, would "follow" our patients. This meant that we would see them on rounds every morning and every evening and write our own notes every day in the chart. We would truck on down to the X-ray department with the resident and intern to look at the patient's X-rays with the radiologist, or to Pathology to look at their biopsies with the pathologist. In the lab we might prepare our own slides of the patient's blood, sputum, and urine and examine them ourselves with the microscope, correlating what we identified in the sputum, urine, and blood with the symptoms and signs of the disease we thought the patient had. Sometimes we would watch their surgeries. So it was a learning experience nonpareil, and in its own sad, exhausting, and terrifying way, it was superb.

My first patient, ever, in my whole life, was Beryl. She would give me my first hint that the medicine I'd been learning, all those facts, all those procedures, actually worked, at least sometimes and maybe often. Also that the body and the mind wanted to improve, and would improve, if you just gave them a nudge in the right direction and removed what was in the way.

Beryl came to the hospital at three hundred pounds, a huge mound of flesh, bearded and hoarse-voiced, with cropped white hair. The ambulance drivers transferred her from gurney to bed and then left. She was in the pulmonary ICU, and we watched from behind the glass partition that separated the patients from the nursing station. The intern, I could see, was disgusted by her appearance, especially by her beard, which no one had mentioned in the transfer, and he sent me out to get the history, do the physical, and write the orders.

Beryl was short, huge, and lying on a heap of pillows, gasping for breath.

Why was she here? I asked her, the traditional opening words.

Her husband had died the week before, she got out in a rasping voice. She had watery blue eyes and a blue, very blue, face. She told him, she told him! if they went to the desert it would be the death of them both, and he insisted and they went, and he died.

"That's too bad," I said.

Her little squinty eyes in her massive face stared up at me and filled with tears.

I changed the subject.

Obviously she wasn't going to be able to give me a complete history, and I couldn't do much of a physical examination either, given how sick she was and all the tubes going in and out of her. So I went back to the nursing station and gleaned what I could from the papers she came with. Then I talked to the social worker who knew all about her. Beryl had been sent to us from a psychiatric hospital, the social worker told me, where she'd been committed after her husband died. Her brother-in-law got her committed because she'd threatened her sister-in-law with a hammer. For calling her fat. Also, she drank.

Over the next week I followed Beryl's progress. I went on morning and evening rounds and wrote a note in her chart every day.

I thought she would die. She struggled to breathe, she gasped and coughed for days. Her body developed sores in its folds and the nurse told me that one of them under the huge left arm was oozing. I put on my best imagined doctor's manner, went over to her bed, lifted her arm, took a sample, stained it as I'd been taught, and looked at the slide under the microscope. It was an infection, and we prescribed antibiotics.

Then the intern told me to get an arterial blood gas so we could learn if she was getting enough, but not too much, oxygen. Arterial blood from an artery is much harder to get than venous blood from a vein. The artery is a thick tube that rolls away from the needle, and in a fat arm, it's difficult to find. Plus the needle hurts when it goes in, and this was my very first one. I went over to Beryl's bed determined, but it was hard to do and she kept screaming at me, hoarsely moaning and crying out as I hunted for the artery, poked, lost it, and kept hunting. By the time I did get it, sweat was dripping off me.

At the end of the week, I changed medical teams and Beryl was no longer my patient. But a week after that, as I was going over to see another patient, I passed her sitting in a chair and I didn't even recognize her. She was shaved and had lost weight and was blue no longer.

She smiled up at me. "Haven't seen you for a while."

I was surprised that she remembered me.

"I'm leaving tomorrow. Going home. And I wanted to thank you for taking care of me."

That stopped me in my tracks. All that time—while I was poking her and she was crying out, while I was clumsily examining her body, while I was watching her struggle and push away our oxygen, while I was asking myself, What are we doing to this poor woman?—she'd been aware and even grateful.

What's more, what we had done during those weeks had worked! She was so much better! Our antibiotics had killed the bacteria in her lungs, the way I'd learned in microbiology; the medications for opening up her bronchial tubes had done their job, the way I'd learned in pharmacology; those painful blood gases had let us titrate the oxygen the way I'd learned in physiology. And in the two and half weeks she had gained of life by our treatment and her suffering, she had turned some kind of corner and her complicated mix of mind and body diseases had simplified and resolved. Medicine had removed what was in the way of her thinking and breathing, and she knew it.

She was even thankful for what I had done, and my heart expanded and my eyes filled with tears. She wanted to tell me and did tell me, and in telling me she gave me something I'd never yet had: a glimmer of what medicine might be—not a set of recipes but one of the few places on earth where giving and receiving can happen so profoundly, so easily, and so naturally.

Every morning we went on rounds to see how our patients had done the day before, reexamine them, reevaluate them, and change their orders.

Rounds had been instituted at the beginning of modern medicine, in Paris during its Enlightenment period, when doctors noticed how much they could learn from patients in the hospital. Especially if they correlated the history and physical examination with the patient's course, death, and autopsy. Being French in origin, rounds retained the hierarchy of French aristocracy: The attending physician was the count, the resident was the captain, the interns were knights, and the medical students were foot soldiers. Women medical students were at the back, camp followers, as it were.

The interns would present each patient, his story and physical findings, and it was like tuning in to a soap opera in the middle. Then Dr. Dole, the resident, blond and energetic, would discuss the case and what to do next. The interns wouldn't write anything down, they would just listen, nod, and remember; and then we would walk over to the next patient for the next story. But one morning Dr. Dole went out of his way, walking over to a patient not our own, who was lying in the last bed of the open ward, in the corner by the window. Dr. Dole read the diagnosis to himself and then turned to us. He knew all about the patient and he had something to teach.

The patient was only thirty-two and a father. Two weeks before, he'd been playing baseball with his son. Suddenly he stopped and his hand went up to his forehead, like this. Dr. Dole put his hand up to his own forehead and winced. He had the worst headache of his life, he said to his son, and then fell to the ground with a brain aneurism that had exploded, causing a subarachnoid hemorrhage. Neurosurgery had operated and stopped the bleeding, but the patient hadn't woken up yet and probably never would.

All of us stood there and looked at the man in the bed, unmoving. We were all young. We all played ball.

"One of my best friends had a subarachnoid hemorrhage," Dr. Dole continued. "We were interns. He was two months married. Good guy, great doc. He was rounding with his team and suddenly put his hand to his forehead, like this." He showed us again. "And said, 'Oh my god, this is the worst headache of my life.' Then he fell to the floor and died."

"Right there?"

"Yep. Right there, in front of his patients."

We were all very quiet.

It was at that moment that I saw through the nonchalance of medicine, its coolness, its calm. Here we were, dealing with whatever happens, not in spite of but because we got to experience, here, on a Wednesday morning, in that nowhere hospital at the corner of freeway and mall, the Last Things—Life, Death, Heaven, Hell, Purgatory, and Judgment. Which was why we did it—for our own sakes, to experience the essence of Life, which is that you can die at any moment, suddenly put your hand to your forehead with the worst headache of your life.

As a diversion to what medicine was turning out to be like, I would sometimes sneak off to the little library on campus.

The medical library was an afterthought. It was in a separate building on the second floor, just one big room lined with books and medical journals, with a wooden table in the middle. I would go there to be alone, to explore, and to smell books and paper. One day I pulled out a dusty book from a shelf, bound in leather with gold trim, *Plastic Surgery of the Face* by Harold Gillies, 1920.

I opened it. I stood there for quite a while, turning the pages. Old photographs, black-and-white, staged, portraits really.

You don't see photographs like that, ever, not even today. They were D. H. Lawrence and the Lost Generation come to life. Photo after photo of men with faces blown off in the trenches of the war to end all wars, with no chins, no noses, no eye sockets. Some of the faces were just flat, as if erased. Others had their beautiful young eyes intact, with nothing below, no mouth, no jaw.

The courageous man who wrote the book, I read in the introduction, was a surgeon, and the first doctor to try to restore something to those ex-handsome young men. He took blobs of flesh from the arm, abdomen, or thigh, and then shaped a finer blob to make a kind of nose, a kind of mouth. He wrote about the surgeries, the sufferings of his brave patients, and he showed the post-op photos of his successes, which were almost as bad and in some ways worse than the before, because they were more human and therefore more monstrous. War and what it led to, I learned from that book, might not only be terrible suffering and wasted life but also marvelous medical advances.

So it encapsulated for me the evil and the good of modernity, which was what I was learning—the remarkable advances of what I would later call Fast Medicine.

My rock turned out to be Dr. Greg, who was the attending physician for my final month on Medicine. Tall and white-haired, he was a perfect specimen of the type, in a starched white coat, starched white shirt, and gray silk tie. He was portly, courteous, and fatherly, not part of the competitive brotherhood of residents, interns, and medical students.

Attendings came for one month a year, Mondays and Wednesdays at ten a.m. Sometimes they also stopped by at five p.m. So I would meet Dr. Greg only a few times, but he taught me three things. First, that it was possible, even right, to disobey the law for the benefit of your patient. Second, that it was possible for a man not to be sexist, or, another way of saying it, he treated me like a medical student who just happened to be a woman. And third, that every time we do something to a patient, we also undo something, which would be a Slow insight.

On this particular late afternoon, it was after rounds and I found myself in front of the elevator with him. It was getting dark.

"Let me walk you to your car," Dr. Greg offered.

"Thanks," I said.

The elevator door opened and there were a few people inside. Together we stepped in, and as it went down, he said to me, "I'm going over now to pull the plug on an old patient of mine."

I was shocked.

It was so bold! Code Blues and ventilators were the newest thing, and a counterreaction to them was only just then beginning. There were as yet no "Advanced Life Directives" or living wills, and the comatose patient kept alive with machines was only starting to be seen as a problem. But Dr. Greg was so nonchalant! And there were other people in the elevator! And I was only a medical student!

Did he mean "pull the plug" metaphorically? I asked.

No. He meant in fact.

"He's been my patient for a long time; he has emphysema. There's not much left of his lungs. They're honeycombed and expanded, and on a good day he has trouble getting enough oxygen. In the past he told me clearly that he didn't want to be kept alive with tubes. But I had to put him on a ventilator to get him through this pneumonia. Now he's cleared but we can't get him off the vent. He doesn't want to live like that. So now I'm going over to his room to trip on the cord."

We stepped out of the elevator and headed for the parking lot.

"My daughter is a black belt in karate," he told me by the by as we walked. "She's about your size. A few months ago, she was attacked in a parking lot. She threw the guy on the ground, broke both his legs, and then called the police."

We got to my car and he waited until I got in and the car safely started. Then he walked back to the hospital to trip on that cord.

Naturally, the next week when Dr. Greg came for rounds, I made sure to walk with him to the elevator afterward. And as we waited for it to arrive I asked him: Did he have any words of wisdom for me, a medical student?

The door of the elevator opened and he stepped in. But he held it open for a moment.

"We doctors think we're so important," he told me, "but the way it works is that in any disease about a third of the patients get better, a third get worse, and a third stay the same—and all we do is change who does what."

Then he let go of the elevator door and it closed and I never saw him again. But his words would resonate with me for the rest of my life. They were so strange. Was it true that everything gets better or worse or stays the same one-third of the time, and all we doctors do is change who does what? Dr. Greg was not the kind of person to steer me wrong.

So I began to pay attention.

What I especially paid attention to were the studies of new medications and technologies that would come out every week in *The New England Journal of Medicine*, the premier journal for internal medicine. Every study had a "placebo" set of patients who did *not* get the new medication or technology—so, a Dr. Greg set, which you could compare with the set who did get the new medication. I grew to love that placebo set, and I've kept track of its results to this day. What it has shown me is that Dr. Greg was right. If we look at the good effects of any new medication or treatment, and then make sure to also add in its ill effects—its adverse reactions and side effects—almost every time, it is a wash. The new medication simply changes who does what. It decreases the problem for which it is prescribed but causes other problems, and it ends up about a third, a third, a third.

Of course, sometimes that's worth it. The good effects of a medicine may be better than its bad effects are bad. Chemotherapy, for instance. You accept your 40 percent chance of diarrhea, 20 percent chance of a rash, 10 percent chance of bone marrow suppression in order to get that 12 percent chance of improved survival, or even cure, above the placebo group.

Amazing medications and technologies do come along, of course. Real medical advances have led to real improvements in health, in cures, in lives saved. Beryl, for example. Although we had no placebo-Beryl to compare her with, and she did have side effects from the technologies that saved her life, still, her life was saved. Without the ICU, she most probably would not have survived to give me that thank-you that brought tears to my eyes.

Dr. Greg was counseling me to be not a therapeutic nihilist but rather a therapeutic skeptic. Not every new treatment, medication, or procedure is the miracle drug, the incredible advance that its marketing trumpets. Sometimes it is and sometimes it isn't. It takes judgment to decide whether a new medication is worth it; it takes a placebo group, and it takes skepticism.

So Dr. Greg modeled for me what today I would call a Slow Medicine doctor. He was knowledgeable, thoughtful, and courteous, warm but not intimate, consistent, and reliable. He knew his patient so well that when the time came he did not have to go to the bedside of his now in extremis patient to discuss his Advanced Life Directives. Dr. Greg had already discussed the End with his patient before he got sick, and he knew what his patient wanted, really. His thinking was crisp, which was why he was not sexist. Gender was not a significant characteristic for a medical student, he estimated, and therefore he didn't see it.

And last, and in some ways most important, Dr. Greg was skeptical, from *skeptomai*—to observe carefully, while taking account of the limitations of your observing. You can see only what is possible to see around you, not what is behind you, what is locked in a closet, what just hasn't shown up yet because she works during the day and can't get to the hospital to see her daughter until the evening.

Marcela's mother, for instance.

FIVE

A Successful Petition to the Saint of Impossible Causes

I met Marcela in my rotation on Pediatrics, which turned out to be a lot like Medicine but simpler. Its patients did not have telephone-book-size charts; they did not have complicated families or substance abuse issues. They didn't have many small problems adding up to one complicated hospitalization. They had just one big problem, which it was up to us to find out and treat, if we could.

As on Medicine, I was on a team of resident and interns and we made rounds morning and evening. But it felt lighter. Pediatricians wore bow ties and made balloon dolls out of rubber gloves for their patients. Parents—young, worried, vigorous—were always about. The nurses dressed in bright colors and our patients were sometimes even cured.

Or perhaps it felt lighter because I was more confident. By then I knew the basics: how to examine a patient, draw blood, do a spinal tap. I knew how to do the "write-up," with its crisp demarcation into the "history," which is what the patient told me; the "physical examination," which is what I discovered with my exam; the labs and X-rays; and last, the diagnosis, the treatment, and the plan. It was elegant. It was a story you didn't make up. I particularly liked the distinction we learned to make between subjective and objective, between what the patient said he felt and what we elicited when we touched his body. They weren't always the same.

The piece of the write-up that still baffled me, however, was the "differential diagnosis." This is the list of what the patient might have— all the possibilities, whether likely or not. For instance, if a patient is anemic and vomiting blood, you do not write, simply and straightforwardly: "Anemia secondary to blood loss." Instead you list all the progressively less likely possibilities as "rule-outs," and the longer your list, the better doctor you are. So: "Anemia, rule out thalassemia, rule out hemolysis, rule out bone marrow failure." Why not just write what the patient had? I wondered.

The differential diagnosis seemed precious to me, unnecessary.

Until Marcela.

Marcela Hernandez was smaller than she should have been for her age, which was twelve, and her ethnic group, which was Hispanic, and at the beginning of the week she was admitted to Pediatrics because her kidneys weren't working properly. In those days we could do that: admit someone to the hospital to figure out what was wrong, all at once; get all the relevant tests, X-rays, and consultations; and come up with a diagnosis and treatment in a few days. Kidneys not working properly— incipient renal failure—is rare in children, and everyone was worried and everyone was puzzled.

So at seven each morning, her team would gather around her bed. The intern would summarize what we'd learned the day before: the tests, the consultations, and the state of her kidney function. The resident would listen and give new orders. Marcela would look at us and listen. She was delicate and skinny, with thin arms and legs, straight brown hair to her waist, and big brown eyes. She spoke English but she was shy and never said anything.

At five-thirty p.m. we would come around again and discuss her case once more. Although she wasn't one of my patients, every morning and every evening I would hear the results of her tests, and still after three days in the hospital, the reason for her kidney's incipient failure remained a mystery.

Like any organ failure, kidney failure is a disaster, but it is such a special disaster that we have two kidneys, just in case. Their purpose is manifold. They manage blood pressure. They filter out the waste products our body produces every day from its own metabolism, especially urea, from the amino acids of used-up proteins. They manage the critical balance of salt and water, and acid and base. They produce the hormone necessary for bone marrow to make red blood cells, and they put the finishing touch on vitamin D so it can be used by the body.

So when the kidneys fail, the body entire begins to fail. In the blood, urea increases to toxic levels and acts as a sedative, and a patient in kidney failure will become confused and sleepy. Because of the imbalance between sodium and potassium, acid and base, molecular processes inside the cell begin to go wrong. Because water and salt cannot be excreted, the legs, abdomen, arms, and face swell; the lungs become waterlogged and the patient short of breath. The blood pressure gets very high. The patient becomes anemic and weak, and kidney failure is yet another possibility in the differential diagnosis of anemia.

Medicine's original treatment for kidney failure was "Slow." All the doctor was able to do was manipulate his patient's environment, the "non-naturals," as they had been called in the Middle Ages—the patient's food and drink, rest and activity. So to minimize the urea, the doctor would put the patient on a protein-restricted diet; to manage the balance of salt and water, on a salt-restricted, potassium-restricted, water-restricted diet; for the very high blood pressure, he would prescribe blood-pressure medications; and for the anemia, he would give transfusions. Despite all this effort, however, the patient would continue to feel terrible—weak, nauseated, short of breath. But there was nothing else to do.

Then, about a decade before I met Marcela, Fast Medicine came through with dialysis, at first called the "artificial kidney." It was a machine that could filter the patient's blood, so removing urea and balancing the sodium, potassium, and water. It wasn't perfect; it had a lot of side effects; it didn't treat the anemia; but patients did feel better with it. For children, however, dialysis was still experimental at the time and the team was hoping to avoid it.

At the end of the week, on Friday morning, we all gathered around her bed and the resident went over everything we'd found out so far in terms of diagnosis. That was, after all, the main thing. Only if we had the right diagnosis could we provide the right treatment. Then in a logical, step-by-step way, for his own clarity of mind and also for the benefit of us students, he went over what we knew.

There were three general causes of renal insufficiency, he reminded us—pre-renal, post-renal, and renal. "Pre-renal" meant that there was a problem with blood getting to the kidney. So if the heart or liver was damaged or the arteries to the kidneys were blocked, that led to pre-renal kidney malfunction. Marcela's heart, liver, and blood vessels were all fine, however. We had, therefore, ruled out pre-renal causes for her kidney problem, and we could cross those diagnoses off our list.

Next were the "renal" causes of kidney insufficiency—some systemic process damaging both kidneys—infection, inflammation, cancer. So far, all those tests were negative. But Marcela hadn't yet had a kidney biopsy, and "renal" was still a possibility.

Last were the "post-renal" causes, when the kidneys were fine but the excretion of the urine they produced was blocked by something in the tubes that take urine into and out of the bladder. That is what we are looking for today, he told us. It would be very unusual in a child. It was the elderly who developed the kidney stones and tumors that led to post-renal kidney failure. But that was "in the differential" and we would, therefore, rule it out. So today Marcela would have a cystoscope placed in her urethra to look for stones, tumors, and other blockages.

As he spoke, Marcela listened with the rest of us. She was alone. Her mother would come by in the evening, after work.

That afternoon, the results of Marcela's cystoscopy came back and went around the hospital. That was it! Post-renal! She had some kind of tumor growing right where the bladder drains into the urethra. It had partially blocked the output of urine, and pressure had built up from bladder to ureters and then into her kidneys, which had therefore begun to shut down.

But what could the tumor be? Given her age, nothing good—some terrible, untreatable cancer, most likely. A biopsy had been taken, and now everyone was staying late, waiting around for the pathologist's reading.

At eight-thirty p.m., the report came in. Wow! Everyone was amazed. Proud. We got it! The diagnosis! It wasn't cancer but a neurofibroma, so a benign tumor, which was good, because once it was removed, Marcela's kidneys would most likely recover, and she would not need dialysis. But it was also bad, because the only diagnosis in the differential diagnosis of neurofibroma of the bladder was neurofibromatosis—elephant man's disease. And this was a truly terrible diagnosis.

The disease is caused, we know now, by a deformed or missing protein called neurofibrin, which normally puts the brake on the growth of "things" in the body—tumors, cysts, lumps, and bumps. When the protein is ineffective or absent, as in those with neurofibromatosis, tumors grow everywhere, not only in the bladder but also in the bones, muscles, skin, and even brain. Usually they are not cancerous, but they can still do a lot of harm, causing seizures, bone pain, nerve damage. They also appear on the skin, and there's no stopping them, so the body and, worst of all, the face become distorted, hideous, monstrous. Plus neuro-fibromatosis is autosomal dominant, which meant that if Marcela had children, they would have a 50 percent chance of having it, too.

By this time it was nine p.m. and my resident told me to sit with Marcela until her mother showed up, so he could explain to her what we'd found. I hadn't stayed that late in the hospital very often, and it was the first time I recognized a feeling I would come to know well. During the day the hospital was busy, noisy, with the energy not of sickness but of health—so many nurses, doctors, administrators, so much bustle, so much worry, anxiety, vitality. But when night fell and everyone left for their lives outside, the hospital got quiet, existential. What remained was sadness unalloyed.

I was sitting next to Marcela, facing the doorway, when her mother finally appeared. She was in shadow at first, then a gradually increasing presence, then a kind of hulking and then, as she came through the doorway into the light, I could see—there were things all over her face and neck! Sprouty things. As she came closer, I saw that she was covered—covered!—like the photographs in the textbook I'd just been looking at—with neurofibromas. Her brown hair was longish, drab, and oily, she looked tired, and hanging from her face were dozens of polyps, lumps, cysts. They hung from her nose, her eyelids, her armpits, her neck.

Marcela's mother had neurofibromatosis.

Imagine.

All that effort, intelligence, and expense to get that brilliant rare diagnosis of which we had been so proud, and all it had needed was one look at Mrs. Hernandez.

I went and got my resident and told him, and he kept an unsurprised face when he saw Mrs. Hernandez. He sat down and began to explain and I took my things and went home. But I never forgot Marcela and that experience of seeing the diagnosis develop, almost like an old-fashioned photograph, right in front of me, as her mother came into the light.

With Marcela I saw the power of what I would later call Fast Medicine—of its style, which is technical and methodical, and the pitfall of its style, which is missing the obvious.

That one look at an actual person should have sufficed for the right diagnosis tickled my sense of irony. But it was also a warning: Don't miss the obvious. Back then it was humiliating to miss the obvious. We took pride in our craft, and for a doctor that meant getting the diagnosis right. The best doctor was the best diagnostician. Our attendings embodied that idea by their starched white coats and by their hands— clean, nails clipped, finely muscled, warm and dry. When they shook your hand, it was with just the right amount of pressure for who you were. It was friendly, comforting, and enclosing. You would never suspect that handshake was also for diagnosis.

And with Marcela, we had missed it. True, differential diagnosis had walked us down the correct path, from prerenal, to renal, to postrenal, and there the diagnosis was. So it wasn't a misdiagnosis but it was a missed diagnosis, at least for longer than it should have been. After all, Marcela's mother visited every evening. Someone—a nurse or an intern— must have seen her. Why didn't anyone make the connection? Or the history: Didn't anyone ask about other medical problems in the family? Or the physical examination: Why hadn't anyone picked it up when Marcela was examined? Although neurofibromas start growing after puberty, at least one had grown big enough to cause kidney problems, so there must have been others. It should not have taken a week and all those expensive and painful tests to get the diagnosis. So although Fast Medicine, with its differential diagnosis and its technology, had in the end arrived at the right diagnosis, everyone felt a bit bad. They couldn't take credit for stumbling on the correct diagnosis, and there was a kind of cringe on the part of my intern, my resident, and my attending.

That was the second insight I got from Marcela. There was a pride in differential diagnosis and also a potential for disgrace, even if no one else ever knew.

I would see this clearly a few years later when I was a resident myself. One late night I was called by the doctor in the emergency room to come down and admit yet another patient. On the phone, the ER doctor, Dr. Dobbins, was cavalier. It was a straightforward admission to Medicine: "Little Old Lady—can't walk."

I went down to the emergency room. Dr. Dobbins, big and burly, with thinning hair and acne scars on his face, was relieved to be transferring the patient to me with so little work on his part.

"What's the problem?" I asked.

"LOL, can't walk, room two."

"Any more information?"

He smiled. "Hey, let me know what you find."

Room 2. LOL. Can't walk. I found her. She was alone in the room, on a gurney, tiny and flat under the sheets. Her eyes were closed and she didn't answer my questions, so I went ahead with my exam. I started by throwing back the covers, and . . .

Her right ankle was fractured. It was swollen, twisted, and bruised, and there was bone coming through the skin. No wonder she couldn't walk. This—happily for her and also for me—made her a surgical, not a medical, case. I went back to Dr. Dobbins.

"It's not medical," I said. "It's orthopedics. She has a compound fracture of her right tibia."

Dr. Dobbins cringed.

It's the cringe that's important. That cringe was a good thing, a sign that getting the right diagnosis mattered to Dr. Dobbins; that he took not getting the right diagnosis personally. And that was what I learned about when Marcela's diagnosis went around the hospital. There was a cringe. We had missed it.

Later I would watch the cringe disappear. At first, when I became an attending myself and made a diagnosis that had been missed, I'd call the other attendings and let them know the diagnosis, as I wanted others to do for me. How else would we learn? And for years, there was that cringe, even on the phone, followed by a thank-you and a discussion of how the diagnosis had not been made. It was collegial, helpful. We were all in this together.

And then it began to change. On the phone I could hear a shrug.

"What do you want from me?" the resident would ask. "Do you want me to readmit her?"

This intermediate stage of guilt was followed by a stage of rushed exasperation, as in "Why are you bothering me? I'm providing health-care as fast as I can!"

Marcela's weeklong hospitalization, her series of painful and expensive tests for a diagnosis that should have been made much sooner, went around the hospital, and we all took notice. We didn't want that to happen to us. It wasn't guilt; she hadn't been hurt by the delay. It was shame. And, as the anthropologists have shown, shame is more efficient than guilt. Longer lasting, less angry, healthier.

That cringe was another thing that would disappear when Medicine turned into Healthcare—another piece left out—and its disappearance would be the sign of the victory of Factory over Craft. The shame of a missed diagnosis leached out of medicine, along with its cause, which is its opposite—Pride, the Seventh Vice, the head of them all, which goeth before a fall, but which, as it turns out, is also a virtue, a life-saving virtue.

That cringe is the emotional underpinning of good medicine, of Slow Medicine.

I got one more insight from Marcela. And that was the understanding that there is a whole piece of my patient I'll never know. Surrounding each is a kind of clearing inside of which, invisible, are all these experiences—genetics, environment, their whole life, their families' lives—passed down and through them, appearing on their mother's face though not visible on their own, but autosomal dominant nonetheless.

I could try my best, but I'd never see more of my patient than that fish nostril coming up and breathing the air for a second. I had to be quick, alert, and observant. My biggest strength, therefore, would be to recognize that whatever I saw was only a part. So when something didn't fit, didn't make sense, that was important. Because somehow, with one more piece of data, one more observation, one shift of the frame of my vision, it would make sense.

But it would be Joey Canaan who would introduce me to a whole other realm of not knowing—of not knowing what you didn't know, of thinking you did know—the course of a disease, or the Way of the Newtonian world, and then seeing that sometimes things don't happen that way.

I met him the day we were making rounds with the pediatric fellow, Dr. Nidra. The "fellow" was not quite the same thing as the resident or the attending; neither elder brother nor father, he was more like a visiting uncle—or, in the case of Dr. Nidra, visiting aunt—not responsible for every nitty-gritty thing on every patient, but a warm presence, with more time, and hence able to step back, look at the big picture, take a longer view.

Dr. Nidra wasn't going to be available for rounds the next day, she informed us, because she would be going to pulmonary rounds with Dr. Miller, a lung specialist visiting from Denver. She wanted to ask him about Joey. Perhaps there was something to do they hadn't considered yet, though she didn't think so. They'd already consulted pulmonary and cardiology and Joey was on everything anyone could think of and they still couldn't get him off the ventilator.

Who was Joey? we asked.

Hadn't we heard? It was a terrible story. Joey Canaan. He was three years old, and two months ago he'd ridden his tricycle into the family pool while his mother was in the kitchen. All of a sudden she realized she hadn't heard him for a bit and she ran out into the backyard and there he was, at the bottom of the pool. She screamed for help and the next door neighbor, who was a cop, came running over, pulled Joey out of the pool, and started mouth-to-mouth resuscitation. Then the paramedics arrived and they got his heart going again, but it took them forty-five minutes. So Joey should have had permanent brain damage, but, it was amazing! He didn't. Two hours after he got to the hospital, he opened his eyes, recognized his parents, and was as bright as a button.

"But now he's been in the ICU for two months and we can't get him off that ventilator," she said.

"Why not?"

"Well, normally we wean someone off the vent. We give them breaks, to see if they'll breathe on their own, and we gradually turn down the pressure and decrease the oxygen. But that hasn't worked with Joey because, after two months in the ICU, his lungs have scarred. From the water, and even more from the pressure of the vent, pushing pure oxygen into his lungs. It's not physiologic, obviously. And now, with Joey's lungs scarred, it takes a lot of pressure to push them open. He's just a little boy and every time we stop the vent to let him breathe on his own, he tires out almost immediately, and we have to start it up again. Plus, when we try to decrease the oxygen, his oxygen pressure drops. We just don't know what to do.

"So three days ago, Dr. Hartley, the pulmonary doc, met with the family and decided to try one last thing—a lung biopsy to see if there were any healthy areas left. And yesterday the results came in. In every one, all five from different parts of his lung, there was only scar tissue. So Joey has no lung tissue left, and there's no treatment for that. Dr. Hartley met with the family and explained that it was cruel to keep the little guy going. He'd never get off the vent. He'd never be able to play or breathe on his own, and so Dr. Hartley recommended that if—that is, when—something dramatic happens, we not treat Joey. A Do Not Resuscitate order. A DNR."

"The family agreed?" someone asked.

"Dr. Hartley was crying himself as he wrote it. I'm thinking I'll go talk with Dr. Miller at rounds tomorrow to see if he has any other ideas. But first I'm going to take a look. So far I've just heard about Joey."

We followed her upstairs, down the hall, and through the swinging doors of the ICU to see for ourselves. Joey was in a glassed-in room at the end.

We looked through the window. He had tousled blond hair, big deep-blue eyes. He looked back at us with curiosity. He wasn't scared. He looked like any other blond, blue-eyed three-year-old, waiting until the next thing happened, trusting the grown-ups to take care of things. We watched him for a while. His DNR order was not up yet but would be soon. Every four seconds we heard a whoosh; the ventilator pump moved down, pushing pure oxygen into his lungs, and his chest expanded.

Then Dr. Nidra told us something else. After the meeting yesterday with Dr. Hartley, Joey's father had gone on television and asked everyone to pray for Joey, and the family had a candle lit for him at the altar of Saint Jude, the patron saint of impossible causes. And churches all over the county *were* praying for him.

As it turned out, Dr. Nidra did show up for rounds the next day and with Dr. Miller, the pulmonary specialist from Denver, in tow.

Dr. Miller was not prepossessing. He was overweight and losing his hair, dressed in a polyester shirt without a tie. He didn't do much. He just stood at the foot of Joey's bed and watched. Then he took the chart and began going through the day-by-day and hour-by-hour vent settings for the last, I don't know, months. Then he asked Dr. Nidra to go over everything they'd tried. Increasing the rate but decreasing the volume, the opposite, both at once. He listened to her with his head down. Then he went over to the vent and fussed.

That evening the DNR went up over Joey's bed.

Dr. Miller was at the hospital for the next week, and every morning he came by and fiddled with those vent settings. And by the time Dr. Miller left, Joey was unexpectedly the tiniest bit better. On a little less oxygen, able to take a few breaths on his own. Although, Dr. Hartley explained to Joey's parents, this would not make a difference. With his lungs scarred and fibrotic, he would always be tethered to a machine, with round-the-clock nursing, until sooner rather than later he got pneumonia.

The morning he left, Dr. Miller told Dr. Nidra what to do. Keep going down on the pressure and the volume, but *slowly*. Take your time.

Dr. Nidra followed his instructions meticulously, and gradually she was able to turn down the vent settings. By the end of the second week, Joey was beginning to breathe on his own. By the end of the third week, she was able to turn off the vent and his breathing tube came out.

Without the tube, Joey could talk and eat, and he started to gain weight and strength. His parents brought in trains and trucks and he played with them, and after two more weeks, Dr. Nidra was able to turn off his round-the-clock oxygen. He seemed to be—perhaps not fine but good enough to be completely puzzling. The biopsy had been unequivocal: Joey's lungs were end-stage fibrotic.

By the sixth week there was no reason to keep him in the hospital, and Dr. Hartley discharged him home with oxygen and twenty-four-hour nursing. But within two days it was clear he didn't need the oxygen or the nurses. Dr. Hartley himself went over to the house to make sure, played with Joey, and then sent the nurses and oxygen away.

By Christmas, Joey was riding his tricycle and was interviewed by the local paper.

I heard through the grapevine that after Christmas Dr. Hartley had a copy made of Joey's DNR and hung it up in his office along with a photo of Joey riding his tricycle. And I've always wondered why. As a reminder? Of what? Call in an expert? Never lose hope? When all else fails, pray?

For me as a medical student, Joey was about the *hubris* of medicine—about ignoring the gods, ignoring everything that doesn't fit your scheme, your worldview. For our technological age, that means ignoring or explaining away what we can't understand, what isn't rational, what doesn't make sense, even if it occurs. Joey was the moment I became convinced that modern medicine, technological medicine, Fast Medicine, was amazing but it wasn't always enough—that, despite its power, it wasn't always right.

Joey hinted that there was more to healing than technology. Medicine almost failed him not in spite of but because of its own rationality, its own method. Dr. Hartley had taken enough biopsies to prove that Joey's lungs were ruined, and Dr. Hartley was a smart doctor and a good man. When those biopsy specimens all came back fibrotic, it was rational for him to believe that Joey's lungs were destroyed and that a DNR was the right thing to prescribe.

He was wrong, and it didn't enter his head that he could be wrong.

And just as Dr. Greg taught me to know what I didn't know, and Marcela that sometimes I wouldn't even know what I didn't know, Joey taught me there was more to be known in heaven and earth than is dreamt of in our philosophies. Such as prayer. Prayer worked, at least that once and maybe sometimes and maybe always.

How it works, who knows? It changes the tempo somehow, bends space-time perhaps, so that instead of things going one way, they go another. Or it makes people more attentive, starts a basso continuo in the background that tunes our seventh sense of awareness—even if you're not the one doing the praying, simply a bystander, two people removed.

What struck me most was not the praying per se but its effect. After all, Joey had been in the hospital for two months. Why did Dr. Nidra go see him just then? She went out of her way physically; she went out of her way temperamentally. In part, she went out of her way because of the prayer and the TV. There was suddenly something extra, a jolt. Maybe she went home that night and everyone in her family asked her, "Are you taking care of Joey? We just saw his father on TV." Maybe that's why she came to work the next day so determined to do something.

Then expertise, that peculiar mixture of technology and healing, took over.

I watched Dr. Miller watch Joey. He didn't examine him. No ophthalmoscope, no stethoscope. He spent quite a while just looking at Joey being breathed by that machine. Then he fussed—*fussed* as in "dealt with trifles." It was such a little change he made. But it was counterintuitive. Instead of turning up the pressure, he turned it down; instead of turning up the volume, he turned it down. Just a little. But that was enough to reverse the inevitable—to change destiny, fate, God's will.

You could say, retrospectively, that Dr. Miller practiced Fast Medicine and Slow Medicine together. He knew Fast Medicine so well that he could take his time.

And finally there was the effect of time itself. Tincture of time, they used to call it, and it is the time we've left out of our calculations, out of our healthcare.

Only much later would we find out that, unlike most scarred organs, the lungs do heal, even after drowning, even if they are fibrosed, if the patient is supported medically and has enough time. We didn't think so when Joey was in the ICU. We were sure that scarred lungs would not heal. So another lesson to be gotten from Joey, retrospectively, is this: Slow down. The body is amazing. There is so much we don't know about it and its own healing capacity.

I don't believe Joey Canaan's life would have been saved today.

After his lung biopsy, the case manager and palliative care team would have shown up and begun discussing goals of care. Dr. Nidra would never have had the time away from her computer to go upstairs and see a patient who wasn't, really, her patient, nor the extra time to go to those pulmonary rounds and wait around for Dr. Miller. She would have been too busy entering health-care data to prove that she was providing health care according to all the mandated protocols.

And even if she had somehow made the time, and Dr. Miller had come, he would have been required to put on a gown and a mask and gloves, and he would never have gotten close enough to Joey to be able to do what he did, which I didn't know what it was, but it had something to do with his seventh sense.

SIX

The Mantle of Hippocrates

After Joey, suddenly, I became a different kind of medical student, more of a pre-doctor, as it were.

It was the final year of medical school, we were now considered capable of seeing patients on our own, and the school had a long list of clinical electives we could choose from. We could be a "sub-intern" at the biggest county hospital in the country, doing the work of an intern but supervised, with only one or two patients. We could go to Africa and learn public health face-to-face. We could sign up for a rural practice, a private practice, or an inner-city clinic.

My friend Rosalind chose London and neurology, and she loved it. It was so nineteenth century, relying not on technology but on expertise, she would tell me later. Its tools were even more arcane than Craig's—great round rubber hammers for testing the patient's reflexes, a rolling pinwheel for checking sensation—and with them the English neurologists could localize brain lesions almost as precisely as a brain scan. For a century they'd been celebrated for their meticulous exams and their eccentric tools, and they were amazing to watch. Quiet. Observant. Precise. In an hour they could diagnose where in the brain the lesion was, and usually what it was, too, just by the reflexes, movements, and twitches they elicited—although, alas, they had nothing much with which to treat it.

Even more intriguing was their lifestyle. English medicine, Rosalind told me, was not as hectic and rushed as ours. The doctors in England took their time. At eleven a.m. and four p.m. they had tea—not a tea bag in a plastic cup as they ran upstairs or talked on the phone, but brewed tea— milk, please, and two teaspoons of sugar—in the doctors' lounge, where they visited with one another. In the evenings when they were on call, they went to the pub across the street from the hospital. It had a direct line to the emergency room, and if something came up, they would leave their pint, go over, examine and admit their patient, and then return.

I, on the other hand, wanted to see patients who were not as sick as those I'd been seeing. What would it be like, I wondered, to see patients before they fell completely apart? What would it be like to be a doctor in the countryside? In the inner city?

I started with the inner city. Our county offered a free clinic to women for birth control and to men for the sexual diseases that were, in part, the result of birth control, and my first elective was there.

In the Sexually Transmitted Disease Clinic, I saw the breadth, width, and length of sexual practices. It was run by Dr. Vander, yet another gentleman doctor. Tall, white-haired, and quiet, he sat at his desk, listened to the complaint, then swung his chair around so he was eye to eye with . . . the problem. He didn't wear gloves but used two Q-tips to lift up and look at the problem and take cultures. He said little. A few pointed questions. Then he would leave and make a slide and examine the slide himself with the microscope. I would follow him and he would show me. Gonorrhea, syphilis, chancroid, trichomonas . . . It was always something, and he always knew what it was and had the antibiotics to take care of it. And the more ghastly, drippy, and horrifying the venereal condition, the more fastidious he was. He taught me how to listen with interested, uncritical face, then gently but carefully examine those

private parts, taken out of businessmen's slacks and workmen's dunga-
rees with such embarrassment, and how to test and even to identify with
his special microscope the deadly twisting spirochete of syphilis.

Dr. Evans, who ran the Women's Clinic, was Dr. Vander's opposite.
She strode into the exam room, greeted her patient, pulled up the stool,
glanced at her tray, and then fit diaphragms and put in IUDs while
querying the patient in the most efficient way imaginable. Clean, not
messy, and not in a hurry.

There was something remarkable about the two of them. Though Dr.
Evans was fast, trim, and efficient, and Dr. Vander was slow, thoughtful,
and deliberate, they were a matched set. Inside Dr. Evans's Fast was a
kind of Slow, and inside Dr. Vander's Slow was a kind of Fast. Though
she moved briskly, there was no waste of effort or movement, and
though he moved deliberately, he too wasted no time. Efficient but not
hasty, their actions came out of a calmness, a confidence, and an expertise. It was very attractive and I wanted to have it someday.

Medical school was turning out to be very cleverly constructed. It was
built upon and began with a foundation of Fast Medicine—of facts,
experiments, data, and knowledge; then came learning to question the
patient's actual body in front of you, then the finding of the story, and
last of being skeptical, which is really the keeping open a space for
everything you don't (yet) know or that doesn't (yet) fit. And finally,
there was trying out what you'd been taught in all kinds of different
situations. Learning how things really show up, not as fictional cases
where everything is in order, with neat pictures and synthetic data, but
in the gesture of shame and embarrassment as a patient takes his dripping private parts out of pressed slacks, sheepishly revealing, but only
in part, the cause of his symptoms.

For an experience in the countryside, I chose an elective at the Farm-
workers' Clinic. It was in the Central Valley of California, down the

freeway, off a road, on a little street, outside a town. The faculty wives of our medical school provided a stipend of eight dollars a day, which was the first money I earned as a doctor, and a mobile home in the trailer park two blocks from the clinic.

The clinic had two doctors, two nurses, a radiology tech, an X-ray machine, and many patients, all Spanish-speaking and young. I would follow the doctor into the exam room, listen to what he said and watch what he did. You never knew what you were going to see. One woman came in quietly but in full-on labor; we cleared out the waiting room and Dr. Howard delivered the baby right there in the middle of the clinic.

What impressed me most, however, was how he handled the farm-worker who walked in with a nosebleed. It was gushing; the man was holding a rag to his nose and the rag was soaked with blood, which was dripping onto the floor. He was terrified, his blood pressure was very high, and the nearest emergency room was thirty minutes away. I wasn't sure if you could bleed to death from a nosebleed. I didn't think so. But I did know that the patient's terror was part of why his blood pressure was so high, and that his blood pressure being so high made the blood pump out of his nose even faster. Almost everyone was anxious. Blood is scary even if you're a health professional.

But Dr. Howard was calm. He asked the nurses to bring over the clinic's gurney and had the patient get up on it. He started the IV, ordered an ambulance, and then applied pressure to the anterior nasal septum with his fingers. It might take ten minutes to stop the bleeding, he told me, but it would stop. All bleeding stops.

After ten minutes, however, the bleeding hadn't stopped. It was still gushing.

It must be a posterior bleed, Dr. Howard explained. Those were more dangerous than anterior bleeds because they don't respond to pressure, being too far back in the nose and often arterial. What was critical was to get the blood pressure down, but unfortunately the clinic didn't have any rapidly acting IV medication for high blood pressure.

For about a minute he stood there while the patient hemorrhaged around his fingers, the nurses fussed, and I watched him think.

Finally he said to the nurses, "Get me a vial of Thorazine."

Now, Thorazine is an antipsychotic medication that I'd already used in psychiatry, and it comes in an IV form for psychiatric emergencies. Among its side effects are hypotension—lowering the blood pressure—and sedation, and I watched Dr. Howard inject it through the IV, even though he knew the patient was not psychotic. He was using the drug instead for its side effects. And it worked instantly. The patient's blood pressure started coming down and he began to calm down. After two minutes, the nosebleed began to subside, and by the time the ambulance did arrive, it was down to a trickle.

That impressed me. That stayed in my mind. I could use a medication for its side effects—in fact, a side effect was simply another power a medication had. It was a side effect only because of the frame we put it in, its category. That frame—"This is an antipsychotic medication"—was what put its other, possibly handy effects—lowering blood pressure, tranquilizing a patient—to the side. But Dr. Howard had thought outside that frame. He had used Thorazine for its perhaps lifesaving side effects, and he had opened up for me a whole new way of looking at medication.

As I walked back to my trailer that evening, I parsed it out. Thinking the way Dr. Howard thought meant I could use medications for their side effects. So I could use a medication that had "weight gain" as a side effect for a patient who needed to gain weight, or I could use a medication whose side effect was "nausea" as an appetite suppressant. I could use a medication whose side effect was "agitation" for somnolence and a medication whose side effect was "sedation" for insomnia. A medication that caused miscarriage could be used to abort, and a medication whose side effect was eyelash growth could be used to thicken eyelashes.

All those side effects I had learned about in pharmacology were actually powers I could use, and my black bag was more like an artist's palette than I'd realized. Instead of hundreds of medications, in effect I had thousands, and it would be up to me to figure out the best formula for the effects I wanted. From Dr. Howard on, I would always think how I could use medications whose side effects I wanted so that my patient would be taking the fewest number of medications, the most elegant set.

Later I would realize that drug companies know this trick of ours, and for decades they tried to keep track of the "off-label" uses that doctors came up with. That was difficult to do with paper charts and prescriptions, but with electronic health records, it became easy. The drug companies buy that Big Data from the electronic health record (EHR) vendors, and when they find a medication that is often used for a particular side effect, they rebrand it, market it for that new indication, and quintuple its price.

It also drives the algorithm providers crazy, because how can they manage and score what doctors are doing if doctors use antipsychotic medication for hypertension, sedation, or weight gain? How can they keep track? It does not fit their paradigm and they would like to make this off-label use of medications illegal, or at least EHR-impossible. They haven't yet succeeded and I hope they never will, because Dr. Howard's Way is part of what makes Medicine not only a science but also an art.

The best month of medical school, however, turned out to be the last month. It would be the first time that I would realize I might actually like being a doctor.

It was one step further along, not a clerkship nor an elective clerkship but a "sub-internship" with the general practice of Drs. Wellock, Neil, and Grace, and it was in the Wine Country of California. It was a "sub-internship" because, having finished if not graduated from medical school, I would be allowed to see patients on my own.

Everyone said it was impossible any longer to be a general practitioner—there was just too much knowledge, too much information; no one could do it all. But the country practice of Wellock, Neil, and Grace did do it all, and it was open to medical students. We could sign up for four weeks and stay with Dr. Grace and his six children in his big house or, if we preferred, by ourselves in a cabin he owned out in the vineyards. It had no electricity but it did have water, he told me when I arrived, and it was quiet, and I took that. And for the following month I saw patients in his office, went to surgeries, and made house calls with him in his big truck.

It was an eye-opener. He and Dr. Neil had been "gold canes" at the university medical school, and their gold-headed canes, which were really gold and really canes, were given to the best medical student in each graduating class, and on display in their office. Together with Dr. Wellock, they had set up an old-fashioned practice, which was old-fashioned even at the time. Fearless might be a better word. Fearless and bold.

The three of them did everything. They delivered babies and, if necessary, did the C-section. They did their own surgeries and were one another's anesthesiologist. They did their own well-baby checks for the mothers they delivered, and were the pediatricians for the babies as they grew up. They did their own Pap smears, breast exams, breast biopsies, and postsurgical checks. If the biopsy showed cancer, they gave the chemotherapy. If the patient got depressed from the chemotherapy, they were the psychotherapist. They ran their own smoking-cessation programs, taught medical students, and took care of their own patients in the hospital.

And they were happy and satisfied with their lives and their medical practice, or so it seemed to me.

Dr. Grace assigned me my own examining room in his office, and for the first time I saw patients by myself. And I was astonished. I knew—kind of—what I was doing. Medical school had worked!

The patients would come in and they would undress—man, woman, child—sit on the examining table, and tell me what was bothering them. I would ask them questions. I would examine them. And then I would write up my findings and workup, and go out and find Dr. Grace, and tell him what I wanted to do.

And he would say, Right! Go do it! And I would go back into the patient's room and tell the patient and . . . he would do it! Take the medicine, have the test, change his diet. Then he would thank me, shake my hand, look into my eyes, and give me a smile.

It was way better than I'd expected. The patients looked at me with trust, admiration, and confidence. It was different from anything I'd ever experienced.

So toward the end of that month, I decided to ask Dr. Grace about it. We were out in the country, driving in his truck on a dirt road after a follow-up visit to a woman and baby he'd delivered ten days before.

I told him how strange it was. The patients listened to me, revealed themselves to me. They assumed I had some kind of power, wisdom, and they were confident that what I said and did was for their own good.

It was that confidence that I wanted to talk about.

"I'm a small woman," I said to him. "I'm twenty-seven. I'm not even a real doctor yet, and still the patients open their shirts and their hearts and their minds to me and they pretty much do what I tell them to do. They treat me differently from how I've ever been treated. Not only respectfully but with honor—no romance, no trivialization. It's particular."

"It's the Mantle of Hippocrates," Dr. Grace said, his eyes on the road. "When that's put on you, at your graduation, and you have 'MD' after your name—you just wait. You'll be amazed. It changes everything."

"What's the Mantle of Hippocrates?" I asked him.

"It's what happens when you become a doctor. It will be even stronger when they lay that hood on you. After that, for the rest of your life, you'll be treated differently, and you'll be different. When you talk, people will listen—even if you're not talking about medicine but about politics or religion. What you say will carry special weight."

And with that, I was done. Medical school was over.

I hadn't gone to my college graduation, and I went to my high school graduation only because I had to. But medical school graduation was different. Medical school had been hard and I was proud of having made it through. It had required the best of me—and parts of me that weren't my specialty. Patience, for instance. Humility. A kind of clarity and detachment from other people's suffering while still being attuned to it.

So I was proud to go to the ceremony.

It is called a hooding. That Mantle of Hippocrates that Dr. Grace had talked about turned out to be a real mantle, a green velvet hood that originated in the Middle Ages, when the color for the medical degree was green, and only doctors of medicine could wear it. My classmates and I walked into the auditorium, with our families in attendance; we were wearing our black robes and our rented mortarboards. Row by alphabetical row, we stood up and waited for our name to be called.

My name was called and I walked up the stairs onto the stage, where the Dean of Medicine was standing. I was the sixty-seventh student, and yet he still looked serious, was still attentive. He took the hood, the Mantle of Hippocrates, from his assistant, adjusted it, and laid it on my shoulders. It was heavier than I'd imagined. Then he looked into my eyes, took my hand in his, and shook it. His hand was warm, dry, comforting, and enclosing.

And so I had "MD" after my name, the right to prescribe medications and replace my white coat with a stethoscope draped around my neck.

But I didn't yet have my license because, according to Abraham Flexner's 1910 report that has molded medical training until today, four years of medical school are not enough. The graduated medical student needs mentored experience as an intern, where he or she is responsible for patients, but not completely. Since Flexner also believed that the mind was not wholly divorced from the brain, he insisted that even a psychiatrist had to have that experience.

I looked around and found a nearby psychiatry residency at the VA, with an internship of eight months of psychiatry and four months of medicine, and I settled on that.

It would not turn out to be what I expected.

SEVEN

Three Prophets, No Whale

On Thursday afternoon of my first week as a psychiatric resident, I met with my supervisor, Dr. Langley, who would be mentoring me during the year. He was young and long-limbed, sprawled in his chair. He had bushy brown hair and a full brown beard, and if something captured his attention, he would stroke his beard with long meditative strokes.

Theirs was a Freudian-based program, Dr. Langley explained, and I would be meeting with him every week to present my psychiatric patients to him. The patients would be assigned to me as they came in through the emergency room, I would diagnose and treat them, do therapy with them, and prescribe their medications; and if electric shock was needed, I would give it myself. He would advise me on their psychotherapy and their medicines. During the year, I would see all three of psychiatry's main categories—psychosis, neurosis, and personality disorders—and I would learn to distinguish them: the sociopath from the severely depressed, the histrionic from the hysteric, the manic from the schizophrenic.

Then he handed me the keys to the locked ward.

Be careful. Don't get trapped in a corner of the examining room or on the wrong side of a door. Above all, remember: Sometimes it will be hard to tell who is crazy and who is not. I was not crazy, by definition. I was the doctor, on this side of the desk, with the keys. The person sitting over there, on the other side of the desk, was the patient. By definition.

Unlike in medicine, there were no blood tests or X-rays that made these diagnoses for us, he went on. Psychiatry's diagnoses were usually subjective and clinical. Of course some psychoses could have physical causes—drugs, strokes, syphilis—but they were rare and won the patient a bed on Medicine. The others, for which no physical cause could be found, were the psychiatric, and included schizophrenia and the major affective disorders of manic-depression (as it was called then) and involutional melancholia. The definition of *psychosis* was "a serious distortion in the capacity to recognize reality," and it manifested usually by hallucinations and delusions, and a "disturbance of thinking, mood and behavior." It was, Dr. Langley admitted, a rather vague definition, and yet I would find that, on the whole, I would know psychosis when I saw it.

But what about Jung? I asked.

Forget about Jung. Jung was crazy—a psychotic, a schizophrenic.

During the first four months of that internship year I spent a lot of time in the locked area for acutely psychotic patients called the Day Room. It was right out of central casting—a wall of barred windows, a sofa and coffee table with old magazines, television hanging in the corner, and patients sitting in chairs, lying on the sofa, or milling about, talking to themselves.

Since there wasn't much pressure for a quick discharge, I could watch my patients' progress and see how well, or not, my prescriptions were working, and how well, or not, our talk therapy was going. It didn't take long to learn to identify our three main diagnoses—schizophrenia, mania, and depression—and differentiate them from their imposters—drugs, hysteria, and fraud.

Schizophrenia in particular had a characteristic set of symptoms and signs, and in that, and its stereotypic response to medication, it did seem like a disease. Thus the schizophrenic had a way about him that was just about diagnostic. He would be restless and agitated, walk stiffly, touch his hair distractedly. He would be undone—buttons undone, zippers undone, hair uncombed—too excited for all that. He would speak rapidly, and all over the place. He would hear voices, and they would always say the same kinds of things: he was chosen by God or the Devil, he was being followed by the FBI or the KGB; the radio and television had messages for him. Then, after he got antipsychotic medication, these symptoms and signs would begin to disappear. The patient would start buttoning his buttons and zipping his zipper, his speech would slow and connect back up again, the voices would grow faint. He would return to Planet Earth and become "oriented and cooperative," as we learned to write in our notes. So schizophrenia seemed more like a disease than a mental condition; it had a course, a prognosis, and a predictable response to medication—like strep throat.

But there were differences. The schizophrenic did not believe he was sick, and our antipsychotic medications worked only so well. In that, it wasn't like strep throat and penicillin. Our medications did not cure the disease. They subdued the patient and disappeared his voices and often he could be discharged, but it wasn't a cure. At the same time, I noticed, even when the patient was at his worst, his mental fever at its highest, there was still some fundamental wellness in him, as I learned from Mr. Parker.

For weeks I'd been seeing Mr. Parker in the Day Room. He was middle-aged, small, and compact, shaved, but badly; his shirt buttoned, but not perfectly. Every time I unlocked the door, I would see him pacing, stopping at the television for a minute, staring up at it with an anxious expression, then pacing again.

So one day I started pacing along with him, at his side but arm's length, which is important with the schizophrenic—not too close. I walked down the ward with him, we turned, and then started back. He was muttering to himself, shaking his head and wringing his hands.

Finally I asked him, "What are you afraid of, Mr. Parker?"

He looked at me with frightened eyes and shifted his weight from side to side. "I heard on television that Hitler said Europe needs another bloodbath."

"Is Hitler alive, Mr. Parker?"

That took him aback. He thought for a second, and then said, with a smile, "No, no, he's not!" But immediately his face froze up again and resumed its frightened stare.

Just then the lunch bell sounded and Mr. Parker came to a stop, turned, and shuffled off to the dining room. I followed and watched how he, and our schizophrenic murderer, and our slow-moving catatonic, and all our other psychotic patients, took trays, waited in line, and chose the food they wanted. Then they walked over to the table, sat down on chairs, and ate. Each used his fork as a fork and his spoon as a spoon, and they were as quiet and concentrated on eating as anyone.

I found this remarkable. They were all crazy, hallucinating, un-hinged, and terrified, and yet—not for everything. The lunch bell rang and somehow they left their hallucinations in the Day Room. What did it mean about psychosis if its victims could wait in line and eat with knife, fork, and spoon, despite Hitler and his bloodbaths? They weren't always crazy about everything. Somewhere there was health.

I wondered. Perhaps they take, and we take, their hallucinations too seriously. We all hear voices in our heads. We learn to ignore them or hear them as our own voices, though Jung treated them as inner beings independent of himself, which was why the Freudians called him schizophrenic. But what kind of categorization is that? Jung lived a long life, produced stable children and an immense body of brilliant work. Would we really have wanted to cure him of his disease?

Psychiatry turned out to be a civilized internship. We had enough time to sleep, rest, and study; we read and discussed and wrote papers. I did psychotherapy with my patients and had my weekly consultation with Dr. Langley. Often my patients would get better enough to be discharged, although it was an unsatisfying better, a chemical or electric "better" but not a cured better. In a way it was a cured worse. I experienced this for the first time with my patient Mr. Sunshine.

Mr. Sunshine's real name was George Johnston, and he was married, was a security guard, and lived with his wife in a one-bedroom apartment. He was thirty-three years old, and they had a thousand dollars in the bank. Which is to say, he wasn't anybody. And then the Voice of God came unto him and said, "Preach, preach to the heathen, to my people, to repent."

I couldn't tell from talking with him how long it took him to accept his mission; whether he took a metaphorical or even a real boat for Tarshish to escape the Voice or spent three days and three nights in the belly of a fish. I did learn from his wife that she was horrified and thought he was crazy, and that they fought; that he legally changed his name to Mr. Sunshine and then took all their money out of the bank and bought Bibles and business cards and had the Bibles inscribed "With the compliments of Mr. Sunshine." Then he stationed himself on a street corner and gave away a Bible and one dollar to anyone who came by, until he ran out of money and Bibles and his wife called the police.

By the time I met Mr. Sunshine in the emergency room, he was sweaty and none too clean, with a day or two of beard. He looked crazed and desperate but sounded gentle, sad, and confused. He didn't struggle and he didn't have a lot to say. He'd done his best; he'd followed instructions. The county had not repented. His high was turning into a low. Who was he? What had happened to him?

We would admit him and treat him and he would begin to feel better soon, I explained.

He nodded politely, weakly. Would I like his business card?

I would.

He fumbled for a few seconds with his shirt pocket and then extracted a card, crumpled and dirty, and handed it to me.

On thick cream-colored paper, embossed in elegant gray, it said simply:

WITH THE COMPLIMENTS OF MR. SUNSHINE

What a sign of hope, of pride, of election! How lighthearted—how clearheaded—Mr. Sunshine must have felt when he went to the bank and withdrew all his money, smiling at the bank teller; and then to the printing shop to order his business cards. And how happy he must have been, standing on the street corner, handing out God's word and a dollar! And the handshakes, and the smiles of gratitude from all those strangers! Then his boxes of inscribed Bibles getting fewer and fewer, his wallet thinner and thinner, but how thrilled he must have been, despite his wife nagging him as soon as he got home from his street corner every night. She was wrong, he was right: he was elected, and God had chosen him.

Mr. Sunshine turned out to be a very good patient. He took all the medications I prescribed, he went every day to group therapy, and in our individual therapy he was subdued. He didn't talk about voices or prophecy, and in a mere few weeks, he was once again Mr. Johnston, security guard. The social worker telephoned his wife to pick him up, and I saw her, lips compressed and bank account empty, when she arrived. I watched as they went off together, Mr. Johnston, shaved and showered, sparse hair slicked over bald spot, shoulders rounded, in tow.

I was reading not only Freud and Adler at the time but also the antipsychiatrists, R. D. Laing and Thomas Szasz, and their ideas that the mentally ill were simply different, with a gift of sight and hearing, appealed to me. Someone must be channeling God in our culture, I thought, someone must be in touch with the divine and the satanic, and it wasn't anyone I saw around me. Or perhaps what we call mental illness was a fever of the brain or mind—a curative process of dreams and delirium, irrational but still meaningful.

So at my next meeting with Dr. Langley, I asked him what he thought about schizophrenia. Was it a disease? Was it meaningful? Was George Johnston as Mr. Sunshine sick or well?

"Oh," he said, leaning back in his chair, "the schizophrenic talks with God."

"You mean, two thousand years ago in a religious culture they would have been saints?"

"Oh, probably, but I mean what I say—the schizophrenic talks with his God today. For us, sane people who want to talk with God—maybe—we have our ecstatic moments perhaps. But the schizophrenic lives with his God twenty-four hours a day, seven days a week."

What was I to make of that? Dr. Langley was the grown-up, he was the psychiatrist, and even he believed that? Then what were we doing? Why were we treating Mr. Johnston for a disease?

I was beginning to have doubts about psychiatry.

By then the first third of the internship was over, and it was time for me to start the required four months of medicine. As instructed, I stepped out of the elevator on Ward Seven North, the medical floor of the hospital, at 6:55 on Monday morning. My heart sank. With its low ceilings, dim light, and dirty aluminum windows, it felt like Hell. And not Hieronymus Bosch's ironic and colorful Hell either, but a drab, dismal Hell. It was only Purgatory, however—four months.

I looked around for the team but didn't see anyone, so I wandered over to the doctors' office and went in to wait. Its walls were pale green and dirty and it smelled like men's feet. At 7:15, the other intern, be-spectacled, thin, and already depressed, showed up, and then Dr. Dan Kelly, our resident, who would turn out to be a gem.

"Grab a clipboard," he told us, "and a pad of paper, and while we walk around and I introduce you to your new patients, write down what you'll need to do for each one. We have twenty-five patients, so you'll have thirteen," he looked at me, "and you," he looked at the other in-tern, "twelve. Then after you get back to our office, strategize. You'll be tempted to do the easy things first—to whittle your list down to the most difficult things. Don't do that. You'll be here forever, trying to find a spinal tap tray after Central Supply is closed or trying to get a cardiology consult when the cardiologists are all gone. Do what is most urgent first—'urgent' being whatever will keep you in the hospital to-night if you haven't done it during the day."

Though I didn't know it at the time, Dr. Kelly was teaching me a key strategy of Slow Medicine: Do the most important things first and let the others go. It was a corollary to Dr. Greg's 30 percent solution. Be-cause if one-third of patients—and therefore, one-third of things—get better on their own, then by not doing the least important third, you have the best chance of never having to do them. Ipso facto, you save a third of your time and the patient's time and the system's money. You have to stay on top of the non-urgent things, of course, because one-third of them will get worse. But it will take time for them to move up the list in urgency, and when they enter the top of the list, you will catch them and take care of them.

Modern healthcare does not let you do this, which is one of its big-gest flaws. It avoids thinking about problems in order of urgency. Rather, it makes everything equally important, from fastening your seat belt to stopping smoking to having acute chest pain. It is reluctant to judge, and the order it prefers is alphabetical. Dr. Kelly on the contrary took advantage of what I would later know as the "healing power of

Nature": that one-third of things get better over time, and another third don't get worse. You can waste a lot of time on them when the best thing to do is ignore them.

We got our clipboards and Dr. Kelly walked us around the six-bedded rooms, introduced us to our new patients, demonstrated their physical findings, and told us about the staff. Dr. Kelly knew everything and everybody—who was good, who hated doctors, who was vicious and whom we should watch out for.

The nursing assistants would be our allies if we respected them, he told us. They knew a lot and would tell us, if they liked us. But we should always remember that the VA is military. Many of the nurses had been in the army, and all of the patients had been—so, it was "sir" and "ma'am," hierarchy and obedience. Don't ignore that. Use it. You're the doctor, you're at the top, you have authority.

The patients he introduced us to were pretty much like the patients I'd seen as a medical student, with emphysema and cancer, dementia and delirium, diabetes and gangrene. Then we walked back to the doctors' office and Dr. Kelly—"Call me Dan"—explained that the last intern, the one whose patients I was taking over, had vacated the premises ten days before his internship had ended. Decamped. Left and went to Vegas.

How'd he do that?

He just did.

Who'd been taking care of his patients?

No one.

I was amazed. You could leave your patients for ten days and they weren't the worse for wear. In four months I would be done and it was good to know that, worse come to worst, I could leave ten days early. Apparently.

In the meantime, though, I had a long list of things to do because, as Dr. Dan also explained, the most important thing for an intern to do was keep his or her census low. "Census" was how many patients we had, and we admitted new patients when we were on call, which was every fifth day. Sometimes one patient, sometimes ten. There was no limit, which meant you had to discharge an average number every five days. If you didn't, your service would spiral out of control. You wouldn't have time to do the urgent, and your patients would start to "crash"—that is, get sick, with pneumonia, kidney infections, irregular heartbeats. You would spend all your time with your crashing patients but you would still get new patients every fifth night, and your stable patients would begin to "de-tune."

What was that? I asked Dr. Dan.

De-tune is what happens to a complex medical patient if he or she stays too long in the hospital. Maybe he comes in with decompensated heart failure, and you work on that and his heart gets better, but the medications you've used to dry up his lungs also dry up his kidneys, and his incipient kidney failure gets worse and then you have to deal with that. He "de-tunes." So that while the first stage of his stay in the hospital is treating the admitting diagnosis, the second stage, before you can discharge him, is a recalibrating, a retuning of all his other problems. It's subtle, and it has to be slow, because any abrupt changes will evoke the opposite. For instance, rehydrating the kidneys might flood the heart; giving a transfusion to treat the anemia caused by chronic blood-drawing might cause chest pain. So retuning is an art of going just fast enough.

The third stage, then, is when the patient is finally, once again, "tuned." But not like a car. Like a piano. It is a golden moment. Because if the patient stays longer in the hospital, a day or even sometimes just a few hours longer, he will start, once again, to "de-tune." With a bladder infection or an arrhythmia, a fall, a delirium. Patients can end up staying for weeks "circling the drain."

With those final words of wisdom, Dr. Kelly left. The other intern disappeared, too, and I was alone in the doctors' office. It was ten a.m.

I looked around. The place was filthy. There were tubes of old blood on the desk, a bottle of culture medium growing bacteria in the drawer. Unneeded chairs filled up the space, and there were old charts all over. In the corner was a coat rack bearing the stained white coat, stethoscope, and drooping tie of my vanished predecessor.

I started with the urgent, which was clearly to clean up that room. I would never be able to work with focus until it was straightened out. I took the old call-schedules off the walls and threw out the blood tubes and culture bottle. I cleaned out the desk, moved out the chairs, and piled up the clothes. Then I called plant services. The doctors' office had to be painted STAT. . . . Dr. S, that's who.

Last I stamped up a set of index cards with the names, dates, and serial numbers of my new patients, took my clipboard, and went out to get to know them. If I could have done anything else, I would have. But there was nothing else to do.

The thing about the VA was that it was just competent enough, and everyone was satisfied with things as they were.

The nurses, social workers, and administrators were there for the duration, so don't rock the boat, loose lips sink ships. Their days had a pattern they liked well enough. The patients, too, were pretty satisfied: they had a bed, a sixth of a room, a breakfast tray, lunch tray, and dinner tray.

The nurses had their army years behind them and a pension in front of them, and every year on the first of July a new class of interns would arrive, scared, idealistic, determined to change things. But all they had was one year, and by the middle of the intern year, that is, by Christmas, when the trees came out of their boxes to be dressed in dusty ornaments, the interns, too, began to get the idea. The VA was good enough, and now they had only six months left—five if you didn't count the last month, and why would you count that?

Which is how long it took me, too, to get the idea.

I took Dr. Kelly's advice, which was a Slow Medicine approach when you think about it: Do what's most important first. And by Christmas, I, too, as a medical intern on Ward Seven North, was good enough. I knew how to admit patients and work them up, and I knew how to discharge them, which required even more finesse, since they usually didn't want to go, the nurses didn't want them to go, and, in order to get them to go, all their tests, for each of which there was a long waiting list, had to be completed.

At first, I followed the rules. I filled out the forms for consults and gave them to the ward secretary, who would misplace them for days. Nothing would get done. My census would build up and my patients would begin to fall apart, to de-tune.

Then I started hand-carrying my requisitions to the cardiologists, neurologists, and therapists. We'd see each other person-to-person, face-to-face. We'd chat, and my patients would get their consults and therapies. Radiology, however, required a different strategy because no one was visible to talk to. So I put every patient on the schedule for all the scans. Often he wouldn't need them but a different patient would, and I'd go down to Radiology and swap out one patient for another, getting a same-day scan, a same-day X-ray.

Thus my census stayed manageable.

At Christmas, I had two weeks' vacation, and I traded the week after Christmas to a fellow psychiatry intern in exchange for the last week in June. This was how, in the middle of my medical months, I met my second prophet, Tom Sawyer. And if Mr. Sunshine was the apotheosis of a psychiatric disease that we could palliate but not cure, at least not with chemicals, and that left me almost as sad as he was, Mr. Tom Sawyer would leave me with an emotion altogether different.

Like Mr. Sunshine, Mr. Sawyer had been called by the Lord. In his case, the Lord told him to change his name to Tom Sawyer. His given name was Samuel. But that was what the Lord wanted. The Lord was emphatic. And Samuel obeyed. He legally changed his name to Tom Sawyer.

I never learned what else he did while he was possessed. By the time I saw him in the ER, he didn't seem that crazy. He was slim, with thick brown hair and tight jeans, swarthy and masculine. It was winter, and perhaps he wasn't crazy at all but simply needed a place to stay. Some of the psychiatric patients did make the rounds—Florida in spring, New England in fall, California in winter, riding the rails—and in group therapy, they would pass along tips about which psychiatric hospitals were best. Mr. Sawyer was not agitated, scared, or paranoid; he was pleasant and polite. True, he did have one of the signs of psychosis; he was a bit tangential and circumstantial—and he did talk a lot about the Lord, but it was, after all, Christmas. So he sounded crazy but he didn't seem crazy. He said all the right wrong things—he was being followed, he heard voices, he was a prophet, but there was no freneticism, no falling apart of personality.

That night, therefore, I didn't prescribe any medication, and I never knew if what happened next was crazy-real or crazy-hallucinated. But when I came to see Mr. Sawyer the next morning, he told me he had a present for me. He'd sneaked out of the hospital at midnight and hitch-hiked a hundred miles to Bakersfield, he said, to the County Hospital, where there was a huge evergreen tree on the grounds decorated for Christmas. He climbed it, stole the top ornament, and hitchhiked back. And here it was.

Then he handed me an ornament, a large, glittering Styrofoam ball covered with sequins, fake pearls, rhinestones, and ribbons. I turned it over in my hands. We had no such ornaments on campus. Was it possible?

The vacationing intern came back that afternoon; I handed my week's patients over to her. Most likely she put Mr. Sawyer on antipsychotic medication as, I suppose, I should have. But I just didn't want to. There was something so fresh, so hopeful, about his craziness. Change your name, become someone different. Sneak out of the hospital, hitchhike a hundred miles, climb a tree, steal an ornament, and present it to your doctor in the morning.

That wasn't proper of me. I wasn't supposed to side with my patients.

I remembered what Dr. Langley had told me that first day. I was the doctor, by definition, the one with the keys. But during that internship year, anyone who wasn't depressed did not seem crazy.

I never did learn whether what Tom Sawyer told me was true or not. I think it was probably true. He was just crazy enough, and I kept his ornament for years, along with Mr. Sunshine's business card, to remind me of the power of prophecy.

Then I went back to medicine.

The weeks passed. I grew pretty tired and pretty depressed.

Actually, depressed-tired and tired-depressed. It's a special state that interns get into. Not depressed from the usual causes—reversals, self-insights, ill health—and not tired so much as depleted, a well run dry. The well was life force, ebullience, Whitman's "Sun-rise would kill me / If I could not now and always send sun-rise out of me." It was the state of being no longer able to send sunrise out of you. And the intern is facing a dark night—a fearful nothingness that he or she has never seen before, that society hides away in tall fluorescent-lit boxes. And that he or she has to get through, because there is no other way to be a doctor except to get a medical license, and there is no other way to get a license except to get through.

The Chinese call that life force *chi*—essence—from the steam that floats off just-cooked rice. And around the middle of month seven, the intern's chi is gone. There's nothing left to ward off the weird tension of the hospital, made up of its workers, for whom it is a place of wage earning, gossip, and politics; and its customers, for whom it is a never-before-thought-of place of horror, where legs are cut off, poisons given, and nothingness faced.

By then the intern is in a kind of shock, made up of exhaustion, horror, and meaninglessness. And that is where I was. All I could do was get through. Minute by minute, step by step, patient by patient.

And then. Out of the night that covered me, black as the pit from pole to pole—a turning point.

It was four o'clock in the morning, and I was in the Admitting Ward, examining my next patient, who was in bed, with curtains drawn. The ward was filled with patients but it was quiet, the light dim, the feeling, as it so often is in a hospital late at night, melancholy.

I was absorbed in the thousand details of the physical exam—the skin, the pulse, the obscure story—while in the next bed, the other intern had a very sick patient. I'd seen him as he was rolled in on a gurney. Bloated and blue and still, he would die soon, I could tell. But by then, even death had lost its sting. All it meant for us interns was that we filled out different forms and didn't have to transfer the patient in the morning.

And then, all of a sudden, there was a noise on the ward, a rustle, and I looked around the closed curtain. A priest in black cassock, book in one hand and gold cup in the other, was gliding through the quiet ward, and stopped at the next bed. He went behind the curtain. At first there was nothing, and then I heard a murmur and began to smell incense.

I went back to examining my patient and had just reached his gangrenous toe when suddenly I heard a little bell, high-pitched, three times—*ding-a-ling, ding-a-ling, ding-a-ling.* I looked around the curtain and saw that the priest was holding up the cup and I noticed that the ward had become completely still, as if everyone was holding his breath. Then again I heard the little bell, high-pitched, three times, and instantly everything changed—the whole pitch of that melancholy ward. Because that second ringing meant we were now in the presence of the Coming of Death, and here He was, now, in our midst, in the next bed.

It was my first experience of dying, that rite of passage, and my eyes filled with tears. We were all on that same promontory, I suddenly understood, not intellectually but in my very heart; every patient in every bed in that dim room, the nurses, the doctors, the janitor, and myself; and Medicine was a noble profession. It dealt with the last things, the most important things: Heaven and Hell, but above all, Purgatory—that mountain from which you can look back and down, whose midway position gives meaning to the rest.

My chi didn't come back after that—it wouldn't for many months—but now at least I understood there was an underneath to what we were doing in the hospital. We were running, examining, writing, puncturing, but underneath there was a stillness where, anytime, two might meet.

I was beginning to have second thoughts.

I liked medicine more than I thought I would—what I got to do, be, and see when I was with my patients. There was deciding what was most urgent and then strategizing the most efficient way to get the diagnosis. There was the camaraderie, the sense of being in this together, not as the health-care team beloved of marketing, but as a group of people with a common goal. There were the patients, and the level to which I had to rise, professionally, morally, and ethically, in order to do a good job.

My patients on Medicine touched me. I liked watching them improve, reconstitute, heal. Day by day, their minds clearing, their limbs strengthening, their wounds reconstituting. Not everyone got well, but almost everyone got better, and it was the same pleasure as watching a film go backward. The pieces of the broken vase coming together, jumping back up on the table, the spilled water collecting and running back inside, the tossed flowers righting themselves and reassembling until the vase of flowers is whole again.

And I didn't like what I had to do, be, and see in psychiatry. That peering over my glasses, that distance—doctor on this side of the table, patient on that side. The not-knowing whether what I was doing was a good thing or a bad thing. Was Mr. Sunshine happier as Mr. Johnston? Was Tom Sawyer better back as Samuel?

Jung had not been cold. He didn't take apart his patients, he didn't suffocate their thoughts and feelings under a pharmacologic blanket. He assumed their psychoses and neuroses had meaning; he took his time, he engaged, and many of his patients improved and some were even cured. He even got to the Last Things, but, according to psychiatry, Jung, too, was crazy.

It would be my third prophet, the Prophet of the Avocado Orchard, who would decide me.

It was toward the end of my last months of internship, when I was back on Psychiatry. It was late afternoon and I was called to the emergency room to evaluate a patient who'd been brought in by his father.

First I interviewed the father.

Mark was twenty-five, he told me, and for the past seven years had lived on a rock in an avocado orchard, eating only avocados and reading only the Bhagavad Gita. He, the father, went by once a month to see how Mark was doing, and to try to get him to come home and go to college. But Mark had always refused, until today. Today he went by and Mark got up from his rock, long hair, beard, and all, and agreed to come out. So they got in the car and his father drove him to the ER, because he wanted to know, What did a psychiatrist think? Should he take his son home? Was Mark sane or insane?

Then I met with Mark. He was tall, skinny, and dirty. His hair was brown, matted, and almost to his waist; his beard was long, scraggly, and untended. His shirt was in rags; his bony, pale chest visible; his jeans filthy and falling down his hips. Except for the jeans, he looked like John the Baptist in a Renaissance painting.

He stood in front of my desk and we looked at each other for a few moments, and then he looked down at the floor. I asked him the usual questions. Where was he? What year was it? Was he hallucinating? Was he suicidal? He didn't protest or explain. All he would say was—it was time. The seven years were up and it was time for him to go home, cut his hair, shave his beard, and go to community college.

He had none of the earmarks of schizophrenia. He wasn't agitated, anxious, or restless. He wasn't paranoid or hallucinating, tangential or circumstantial. When I asked him a question, he answered it, or not. He didn't ramble but was quiet and composed. I couldn't tell whether he was sane but he didn't seem to be insane, so I cleared him and out they went, father and son, back to the suburbs and community college. But they left me with a question.

Have we no room for prophets?

Mark was smart enough or resolved enough or mature enough to keep quiet about his visions or voices, and since he didn't talk about them, I didn't have to treat him. But had he talked about them, I would have had to treat him. His disease, if he had a disease, was purely subjective—my subjectivity. As the *DSM* said, and *Harrison's Principles of Internal Medicine* supported, psychosis—schizophrenia—was a clinical diagnosis. Worse, it relied on what the patient said, and whether it was true or not. Hallucinations are only hallucinations if I don't hear them. If a patient is hearing voices through the fillings in his teeth, he is not hallucinating; if he is in fact being followed by the FBI, he is not delusional. And I didn't like that. Medicine was sometimes incorrect, but we pretty much could all agree that there was something wrong with the patient, the patient included.

But in psychiatry, I didn't know any longer what I was treating or what the problem was. Maybe we've drawn too clean a line. Voices and visions on one side; a certain amount of dreaming—but not too much—on the other. But Mark and Tom Sawyer and Mr. Sunshine made me realize I didn't want to be the arbiter.

Jonah was the prophet who tried to escape his destiny, and for him, the whale was the arbiter. After God spoke to him, Jonah took ship for Tarshish, the farthest place away he could think of, and then went down to the hold and fell asleep. Then a huge storm brewed up and the sailors were certain it had something to do with one of the passengers, so they cast lots, and the lot fell to Jonah. So they threw him overboard and he sank to the bottom of the sea, where a whale swallowed him up and then swam for three days and brought him back to Nineveh. After that, Jonah was convinced, and walked into the Great and Corrupt City of Nineveh to announce that Repentance was at hand. And the king listened! The City did change its ways! Turned! *Teshuvah!* A Real Miracle!

Why is this chapter called "Three Prophets, No Whale"?

"Prophets" because as much as Jonah was, Mr. Sunshine and Tom Sawyer and Mark were called to prophesize. As for the whale, I don't know how much each of them struggled before they agreed to prophesize. Perhaps there was a whale and a swallowing and a dark voyage and a vomiting up on the beach of our county. Though I doubt it. Because the whale is the miracle part. Many are called but few are chosen. Many hear the Voice and follow Its commands, I learned on Psychiatry, but the guarantee of Jonah's authenticity is the whale, that big fish who swallowed but did not eat, masticate, or digest him but instead swam three days to deposit him on the banks of Nineveh.

But couldn't my three prophets have had a whale voyage I didn't know about? A three-day Jungian struggle in the belly of the Beast? And prophesized after that, like Jonah?

They could have. That's the point. I could not tell whether they were real prophets or psychotic. The Jungians judge Jung to have been a prophet; the Freudians judge Jung to have been psychotic. The schizophrenic talks with God, even my Freudian supervisor declared.

He also believed that I was the psychiatrist, the doctor, and therefore the judge, the measure of sanity by my own Self. Someone had to be, he told me, but I wasn't so sure. I didn't see a whale; I didn't hear about a whale, but there may have been a whale, nonetheless.

I remembered Mr. Parker, his agitated pacing, how much he suffered, but also how he and everyone else in that locked ward had some healthy, hungry organized place in them as well. I thought about being the person with the keys on this side of the desk. By now we'd read Szasz and Laing as well as Jung and Freud, and I knew of the movement to declare madness non-madness, or socially defined madness. But that wasn't quite right, either. There was something volitional about craziness, something chemical, and something magical. It was a mix.

Psychiatry asked the right questions, I concluded, as my internship ended. What is madness? What is sanity? What is reality and who gets to decide? But it had no good answers. Medicine asked the wrong questions—What is causing that ear pain?—practical questions, not deep and interesting questions. But it did have answers, and I preferred answers to questions. Although, as I realized that late night on the Admitting Ward, medicine itself was founded on the deepest question of all, which gave it standing at the court of my opinion.

And soon I would discover that sometimes even a simple and simplistic question—Why does my son have an ear infection?—could turn out to be deeper than I imagined. Sometimes, though it appeared to be superficial, that question might just be the tip of a Jungian iceberg, the answer to it going deep down into the waters, opening doors, dissolving layers, taking me right in to where people really lived.

EIGHT

Visiting Day at the Henhouse

Since now I had my medical license, I decided to just go out and practice medicine and see whether I liked being a doctor, or not.

I started looking around for a position and a friend of Rosalind's told me about a locum tenens he was doing. *Locum tenens*—holding a place— was a filler position for a physician, he explained. When a medical practice needed a doctor and couldn't find someone to take the position permanently, it hired a locum. The practice provided the office, the patients, the insurance, and all you had to do was show up. The locum he was doing was at a practice owned by three physicians in three separate clinics in California's Central Valley. The hours were eight to six, no night call and no weekends, and you could work as much or as little you wanted. The clinics scheduled the patients, and you were paid a third of what you billed. Anything you couldn't handle you sent to the emergency room.

Could I pull it off with only my internship year behind me?

Well, that's what he was doing. He would mention me to the docs; they had a hard time finding people who wanted to live up there.

At first I worked in all three clinics.

I quickly discovered that outpatient medicine differed from the hospital training I'd received. I didn't have endless time with patients; I didn't have consultants to depend on or an ICU to hand. I saw eighteen to twenty patients a day, and had only fifteen minutes for each one, so I had to focus my history and physical exam without missing anything crucial. It was an art.

The doctors who owned the clinics were good doctors but bad businessmen, and their financial setup was ruinously generous to us locums. They paid us a third of our gross billings, which included not only our visit and anything we did, but also the labs and X-rays we ordered. Since most of the patients were Medicaid patients, and Medicaid reimbursed less than wholesale, often that third was the clinic's entire revenue for the day, sometimes more than its revenue.

For me, it was amazing—a paycheck larger than I needed. It was also morally interesting. At the end of the day, I would check how much I'd billed, and though I didn't order anything a patient didn't need, I wasn't frugal with my ordering, either.

I ended up working exclusively at the clinic in Shafter, a tiny town off the main drag through the Central Valley. It had 7,010 people, with little houses spread out on grids of streets without sidewalks. I liked it best. It was close enough to the County Hospital in Bakersfield that anyone who needed emergency care could go there, but it was far enough away that my patients encouraged me to do whatever I felt comfortable doing.

Other than at the clinic, the only doctor in town was the chiropractor. He'd been there for decades and many patients went to him first. For diagnosis he took full-body X-rays, which were blurry and dark because his machine was old and he used too much radiation. He would hang up the X-ray head-to-toe on the examining room door so it looked like a Halloween prop, and then demonstrate to the patient how crooked his spine was, and what manipulations would be necessary to cure that cough. If he couldn't fix what ailed someone, he sent him to us.

The clinic was small, with a waiting room that was cool and white. Off the hall to the right were four examining rooms and the doctor's office, with a bookcase and a polished wooden desk. Off the hall to the left was an X-ray machine, a treatment room for casting and wound care, and a small laboratory with a microscope and an incubator. The patients were mainly from the Midwest or from Mexico. There were no homeless and no drug abusers, and since the state mental hospitals were still open, no untreated mentally ill. And because Medicaid for indigent adults hadn't yet been rescinded, almost everyone had health insurance.

I saw men and women, the old and the young, and, since the breadth of what I saw was beyond my expertise, I developed a strategy of examining the patient first and then taking his or her chart back to my office and going through it page by page. Thus I would learn which medicines previous doctors had used and for what, and how to work up a symptom. Then I'd write up what I'd seen and take books out of the bookcase to find out more about what the patient had. Every single thing I'd learned in medical school came in handy, no matter that it hadn't fit an overall schema or had seemed pedantic and fussy. Because I'd been exposed to it once, even if I'd gotten it wrong on the test, it was somewhere in my mind and would niggle at me if I saw a patient for whom that "it" might be important. Which was the real reason for having us learn all that detail, I concluded, and all that medical school memorization had been necessary.

The clinic had two staff—Aricela the receptionist, and Kathy the nurse.

Aricela was Mexican American, twenty years old, wore glasses, and had a warm smile. I didn't realize how important she was until she went on vacation and my schedule fell apart. Usually overbooked, I had almost no patients, and finally I asked Kathy why my schedule was so empty.

"Oh, that's because Aricela is out of town."

"How's that?"

"Well, Aricela books the patients, and since she knows them all, she knows when to book them. If you wait too long and book patients too far out, they either get worse and go to the ER, or they get better and cancel their appointments. Her substitute doesn't know that, and she's been booking two weeks out."

Kathy, on the other hand, belonged to the Midwest branch of the Valley's population, although from generations before. Her grandfather had been one of the first doctors in the area, and when she was little, he took her with him on his hospital rounds. She was fine-featured with straight brown hair, and smart, and she loved medicine. Today she would have become not a nurse but a doctor, which would have been a pity because she was an incredible nurse and taught me how to be a doctor. During the year I knew her, she even saved a life.

It was on a Saturday afternoon in Bakersfield and she was walking down the street with a friend when suddenly a body hurled down onto the sidewalk in front of her. Someone had tried to commit suicide by jumping out of a many-story building. He wasn't dead but he had crushed his trachea, and lying there at Kathy's feet, he couldn't breathe through that crushed tube. So she took a penknife out of her purse, stuck it in his neck right below the crush until it reached the trachea, and twisted the blade horizontal. That created an opening to fresh air and the almost-suicide took in a deep breath. But she needed something to keep the hole open until the ambulance came.

Just then the police arrived.

"I need a straw," she demanded of the first cop as soon as he got out of the squad car.

"Sorry, ma'am," he said, "don't have one."

"Yes, you do," she said, with a bit of the convent nun in her, although she was a Seventh-day Adventist. "All cops drink Cokes in their squad car and so do you. Go get the straw out of your drink and bring it over."

He was a big guy in uniform but Kathy was implacable, and he walked over to his squad car and sure enough he did have a Coke in the front seat. He came back with the straw; Kathy slipped it through the hole she'd made in the trachea and kept the guy alive until the ambulance arrived ten minutes later. She didn't even bother to mention her heroism to me—I saw it in the newspaper and asked her about it.

Kathy was the first Seventh-day Adventist I'd ever met. Hers was a very healthy religion, I discovered, and she was a vegetarian and neither smoked nor drank. She didn't not drink because she was an Adventist, though. She just didn't like alcohol, she told me when I asked her one day. She didn't like the taste.

"You should try wine," I said. "It's an acquired taste—I didn't like it at first, and now I do."

"I don't see why I should," she responded. "I didn't have to acquire a taste for chocolate, I liked it right away, and besides, an acquired taste is the hardest to break."

Kathy also had an edge she concealed, an observant, ironic frame for what she saw, and she enjoyed what I enjoyed—the patients, their quirkiness, gentleness, and rapscallion-ness. She didn't like pretension, and no one was more amused than she when the premier cardiologist in town turned out to be a fraud.

It was months into our working relationship. By then we knew each other pretty well; we knew each other's virtues and faults. Kathy's standards were high. She kept the place spotless and organized; fresh coffee was always brewing; whenever we were inside the clinic, she called me Dr. S, and when my white coat was no longer up to her standard, she took it home and brought it back washed, starched, and pressed.

One slow day she stood in the doorway of my office and I asked her about an invitation that a Dr. Dalliwal had sent me, to a Christmas party. Who was he?

Oh, he was the best cardiologist in town, Kathy said. It was almost impossible to get a consultation with him, his waiting list was so long. And every year he gave this big catered Christmas party at his house and invited all the docs in town with their wives, as a kind of thank-you for their referrals over the year. I should absolutely go. I'd meet everyone, and the food alone would be worth it. He had the most beautiful home, the best car, and the most elegant shoes.

Shoes? I asked. I got it about the house and the car, but who cares about shoes? Doctors' shoes should be comfortable. We spend all day on our feet.

I was wrong about that, Kathy told me.

"Shoes are important," she said. "That's how people decide how good a doctor you are," she explained, "by the elegance of your shoes."

That stopped me. My shoes were not elegant. They were shabby, down-at-the-heel shoes. But they were comfortable and I didn't want to buy elegant shoes. I rejected the notion on principle. Appearance shouldn't matter.

"Do my shoes make me look like a bad doctor?" I asked her.

"Well, they do make it harder to see how good a doctor you are," she replied.

That gave me something to think about. My antiauthoritarian Aquarian cohort rejected the accoutrements of power and prestige—the professor's gown, the nurse's cap, the businessman's suit. Excellence would show through, we believed; incompetence would show through, too. Expensive jewelry, stylish haircuts, fancy cars—we preferred the Indian fakirs, who wore nothing at all.

But Kathy was pointing out that I was losing something by that stance, something that was important to me—my patients' confidence. I was putting a stumbling block in front of them, and did I really want to do that?

I didn't go out and buy new shoes, but a few years later at an interview, when I met the attending physician, who was wearing a T-shirt, jeans, a ponytail, and sandals, I myself was taken aback. I had to fight my own inclination to not take him seriously and I remembered what Kathy had said, and went out and bought a pair of expensive shoes. But I wore them only a few times. They weren't comfortable, they distracted my attention from my patients, and they made it harder for me to run upstairs to look at an X-ray. I put them away.

The story of Dr. Dalliwal did not end there, though. Years later, Kathy tracked me down just to tell me so. It turned out he wasn't a cardiologist; he wasn't even a physician. "He didn't even go to medical school!" Kathy told me on the phone.

"But he did most of the cardiac catheterizations in town," I said. "How could he have performed them without any training?"

"Exactly. That's what tripped him up finally. His complication rate was twenty-five percent, and the Medical Board looked into him and couldn't authenticate his fellowship, his residency, or even his medical school."

"How'd he get his license then?"

"Simple. When he applied for it, he told the Board his medical school in India had burned down, taking with it his transcripts and degree."

In spite of this satisfying addition to my side of the ledger, Kathy was still right about those shoes, I thought. Hers was a lesson about the necessity in medicine for form as well as content.

Content is the essence—the knowledge and experience of the doctor, the research and writing skills of the historian. Form is everything else, whatever you see as "appearance" only. The cover of the book, which in theory is "not known by its cover," but which in practice *is* known by its cover; also by its title, its reviewers, its placement in bookstores, and its marketing. Form is everything that appears to be non-essential but that is essential, too. Form is not as important as content; it is, nevertheless, important.

Form means that your patient does not have to overcome a certain reluctance to believe in you. Form means you don't have to un-create the wrong impression. Form is almost free healing power, is what Kathy was teaching me with those shoes. And anything that contributes to healing power should be employed; anything that takes away from it should be abandoned.

I'd never before met people like the people in that little farming town, and I was not only passing them on the street but also seeing them in the most intimate circumstances, in the same room, no more than an arm's length away. They were rarely educated yet they had common sense, and though they didn't have my values, they did have values. It was an introduction to a world I had not known.

There were the men who rode the rails, there was the polluted water that made so many of the patients sickly. There was the Steinbeckian little town itself with a kind of vacant feeling on its streets. The rose-covered houses turned in on themselves, quiet as a Midwestern town in winter, except that all the time—in summer and spring and fall and winter—it was always too hot or too windy, too cold or too wet for anyone to be out. The living room was where everyone lived, on the brown couch in front of the TV, eating TV dinners at twenty-nine cents apiece.

I learned I could not assume literacy and began to draw pictures on the examining-table paper to explain my diagnosis to my patients. When we were done, I would throw the paper away. Then one day a patient asked me if he could have the paper with my drawing on it. And at the next appointment a month later, he took that paper out of his wallet, folded and well worn, and smoothed it out. He had some questions to ask me, and he used the drawing to ask them. That's when I realized he was illiterate, and I began to offer those drawings to my other patients, too.

Also I began to read aloud the directions I was writing on my prescription pad. "You'll take one pill four times a day for ten days.

Make sure you finish the bottle. Don't stop just because you feel better." The patients wouldn't say anything but they would cock their heads and attend. They weren't literate but they were aural.

I learned to speak their language: simple sentences—subject, verb, object. And I learned that I liked them. I admire toughness and clarity and straightforwardness and so I liked them.

They liked me, too, and they accepted me as their physician. Dr. Grace had been right. That MD, that Mantle of Hippocrates, worked, and it didn't hurt either that silk ties were back in fashion for women, and I wore one, along with a button-down shirt, and my man-sized white coat. I would watch my patients' eyes flow from my face down to the tie and the white coat with its MD name tag and then back up, coming to rest on my face with trust. Just to make sure this was not an illusion, now and then I would take off the tie. Without it, despite the white coat and name tag, patients were unsure of who and what I was. With it, they accepted me as that Oslerian third sex, a woman doctor.

I knew for sure I was getting somewhere when, several months into the year, I met Debra's mother.

I came into the exam room and she was sitting on the exam table fully clothed. I washed my hands, dried them, turned to her, and asked her why she was there.

"Hi, Dr. S," she said. "I'm not here for me. There's nothing wrong with me, but I wanted to come in to tell you about my daughter, Debra. You saw her last week."

I didn't remember Debra at first.

"For a throat infection."

"Ah yes. Is something wrong?"

"No, no, she's fine. She took the antibiotics you prescribed and she was better in a couple of days. But a few nights after she met you, I was putting her to bed and she told me she'd decided what she wanted to be when she grew up. I was surprised. We'd never talked about it and she's only ten. So I asked her what it was. What was she going to be? And she said, 'I'm going to be a doctor, Mom, and my name is going to be Dr. Sweet.'"

Then she looked me straight in the face, into my eyes, and we both smiled, a satisfied conspiratorial smile.

But it was Mrs. Laemle who would show me I didn't know anything unless I made a visit.

She came in with her son, Lenny, nine years old, who, she told me, had started shaking his head, picking at his ear, and telling her it hurt.

Now, in medical school I'd learned all about ear infections—external, internal, and middle ear infections; chronic, subacute, and acute; allergic, bacterial, and contact. So I examined Lenny as I'd been taught—not only the bad ear but also the good ear; not only the ear but also the nose and throat and sinuses. The diagnosis was easy. He had a bulging red eardrum. It was bacterial otitis media. I prescribed antibiotics, and told Mrs. L to come back the following week for a recheck. She did. Lenny was better and I signed off.

Three weeks later, however, they were back. Lenny's right ear was hurting him again. I reexamined him, rediagnosed right otitis media, represcribed antibiotics, and rechecked him the next week. Lenny's pain was once again gone, his eardrum back to normal.

Another three weeks and Lenny and Mrs. Laemle were back—with the same problem and the same diagnosis. What was going on? I wondered. Was he not finishing his course of antibiotics? Was the bacteria resistant to them? Did he need to see a specialist?

I decided to try one more time, and prescribed antibiotics once again.

But later in the day I got a call from Mrs. L. She'd forgotten to take the pills with her, and she lived far from the clinic. How bad was it to wait to get them until the morning?

I'd drop them off myself, I told her.

I had an ulterior motive. That morning she'd told me she kept chickens, and I love chickens, and wanted to see them.

She gave me directions to the house—a small house with a chain-link fence. She would wait outside for me.

It was a longer drive than I'd expected, but eventually there it was—chain-link fence, small house, Mrs. L.

In the clinic Mrs. L blended right in, but here, in her apron, with her faded brown hair blown by the wind, she was right out of a photo by Dorothea Lange, only skinnier. And nervous. I was the doctor, after all.

She thanked me for bringing the prescription and asked, did I have time to see the chickens?

I did.

She took me through the gate and around to the back. There was about half an acre of bare dusty ground back there, scrabble in the corners, almost prairie. We walked past a small barn and then stopped in front of a large metal building.

Here's where she kept the chickens.

She unlocked the door and we stepped inside.

It was a huge, windowless space, with a concrete floor, and lit only by a few bulbs strung on a wire across the high ceiling. And it was filled—filled!—with chickens sitting on the ground, walking around. There were feathers everywhere, chicken excrement all over the floor, and up near the ceiling two wooden perches spanned the length of the building, with chickens sitting on them, too. There were cocks abounding, combs gone, tail feathers plucked out, halfheartedly competing with one another in a hoarse, limp cock-a-doodle. The chickens I could make out in the dusk were nearly bald, their wings picked at.

"More'n one thousand chickens," Mrs. L said. "Not many eggs, though. Most of 'em don't lay. But I jes' cain't git mself to kill 'em way I should."

We looked at the chickens in silence for a bit and then we left. She locked the door behind her. On our way back to my car she showed me the pigs.

Now I'd seen pigs before: big fat pink pigs in concrete stalls, with shiny steel troughs. But Mrs. L's pigs were something else again. They were lying outside in manure and trampled straw, covered with flies.

Then we reached the house, and I saw an aboveground swimming pool.

"Them's where my boys go a-swimmin' in the summer," she told me.

We stopped and I stared. There was no filter; the water was still, sitting with scum on top, and it was as filthy as the water in the pigs' trough. I thought about Lenny swimming in that. No wonder he kept getting ear infections. He didn't need an ear specialist; he needed a pool cleaner.

As we walked back to the chain-link gate, we passed a dog in a large fenced area on our left. He was a mutt, skinny, and running in a circle, round and round. We stopped and watched him for a few minutes. He never turned in the other direction and he never stopped.

"Them's Sparks," Mrs. L told me, and shook her head. "Bin hit by a car 'bout eighteen month ago and runnin' roun' like that ever since. Roun' and roun' and roun'. Nothin' we cain do. He won' stop. Probly I should shoot 'im but I jes' haven't got to it yet."

I gave her the paper bag with the antibiotics, and we stood there and watched Sparks run. It was peaceful and awful at the same time. There were the pigs and the chickens, Sparks, and Mrs. L's goodwill and kind heart and slovenliness. There was Lenny and the pool and those recurrent ear infections. There were those little yellow antibiotic pills. As if they could cure what ailed this.

I learned another Slow Medicine lesson that day—that I needed to visit my patients, not necessarily their houses but certainly their minds, their lives, their contexts. I had fifteen minutes to leave my house and enter theirs, realize they couldn't read or didn't have enough to eat, or were very kind. That they were as proud as I was, that as much as I did, each of them lived in their own microcosm, of which they were the center.

But the most important thing I learned that year was what it meant to be a real doctor, and it was Kathy who would teach me.

On this particular day she came into my office at the end of the afternoon to tell me about a patient she'd just put in the examining room. Ed Schumer. The chiropractor had sent him over because he was having chest pain, and I should see him right away.

As I walked down the hall, the possible causes of chest pain went through my mind: the lung causes, the heart causes, the abdominal causes. Most of them were serious, the most serious and most likely being, of course, a heart attack, which we were not set up to manage. Good thing that the County Hospital was only twenty minutes away. I went into the examining room.

Mr. Schumer was sitting on the table, already gowned. He had thinning white hair cut short and growing out over big, flat ears; a grooved and tan face with pale gray eyes; and big workman hands. He was tall and thin, and looked older than his seventy-two years, but he wasn't coughing or short of breath or clutching his chest, which was a good sign. Blood pressure, pulse, respiratory rate were all fine.

The chest pain had started yesterday, he told me. It wasn't a sharp pain, it wasn't a dull pain, he couldn't really describe it. No, it didn't get worse when he took a deep breath, or if he lay down or if he sat up.

When was the last time he saw a doctor?

Six years ago.

I examined him, using that complete top-to-bottom exam Dr. Gurushantih had taught me. Head, eyes, ears, nose, throat—fine. Lungs fine, heart fine, as far as I could tell. Abdomen, arms, legs—no clues. Then I did an EKG. It, too, looked fine, and so after an hour I still didn't know what was causing Mr. Schumer's chest pain. All I did know was that he usually went to the chiropractor, and that he hadn't seen a medical doctor in six years. Therefore, whatever it was—was something.

"I don't know what you have," I told him. "But it's something. You need to go to the emergency room at the County Hospital, where they have heart monitors and consultants and specialized tests, and let them figure it out."

Mr. Schumer's mouth compressed and his eyes were disappointed, but he was a VA kind of guy. He was obedient, he followed orders, and he would go, I knew. I was satisfied that his real problem would be found out, and I went home.

The next day, though, as soon as I came in, Kathy told me that Mr. Schumer was coming back in the afternoon. He'd gone to the ER but been sent home, and now his chest pain was worse.

He looked the same as he did the day before. Blood pressure, pulse, temperature, respiratory rate—the same. He sat on the examining table with the same hangdog look of the day before, he complained of the same pain, he had the same symptoms and non-symptoms. Then he showed me the ER sheet he'd been given. His diagnosis was "bronchitis," and there was a prescription for antibiotics.

That made me mad. Mr. Schumer did not have bronchitis.

I examined him once more. Top to bottom. Hair and scalp and ears and throat and chest and heart and abdomen and . . .

Whoa. I'd examined his abdomen the day before, but I hadn't found this, this pulsating mass, almost five inches across. It wasn't tender, and his liver and spleen were not enlarged. But I was certain that Mr. Schumer had not had this pulsating mass the day before. I walked out of the examining room and found Kathy in the treatment room, where she was reorganizing the bags of IV fluid.

"Hey, Kathy. I found it. Mr. Schumer has an abdominal aneurism, and it wasn't there yesterday."

"He must be dissecting."

"Yep, and that's what's causing his weird chest pain."

An aneurism occurs when there is a weak spot in an artery—in this case, in the aorta, which is the thick, distensible tube that carries your blood from your heart to the rest of your body. Over time, with the blood pressure slamming against it from the heart's contractions, that weak spot—like a weak spot in an inner tube—can start to balloon out, slowly. That's the "aneurism" part. Once in a while that weak place will begin to tear, to split open, from the constant stress of the blood pressure pounding against it once a second, and then the blood inside the artery will start to flow through the tear, to "dissect" it—tearing the tear, as it were. A dissecting aortic aneurism can cause pain, ranging from a mild discomfort to a searing pain, in the chest, in the back, or in the abdomen. The dissection opens the tear even further, which allows even more blood to flow in, and the aneurism begins to balloon out more and more until it suddenly explodes, like a tire exploding. Since the aorta transports all the blood in the body, when it explodes, the patient dies immediately, in a minute.

I went back into the examining room and told Mr. Schumer what I'd found, and explained that it was an emergency. His aorta was tearing apart, and if it blew, he'd die. I drew him a picture on the examining-table paper of his aorta, and the dissection ballooning out, with little marks indicating its incipient explosion.

"That's not what they told me in the emergency room."

"Well, I guess they didn't find it."

"So I have to go back?"

"You do. I'll call an ambulance—"

"No, my wife is in the waiting room. She'll drive me."

A few hours later Kathy called the ER. Yes, Mr. Schumer had shown up, and they'd sent him home once again, with the diagnosis of bronchitis.

She came into my office. It was, by this time, the end of the day.

"I called Mr. Schumer," she told me. "He's back home. I told him he *had* to go back to the ER, but he said, 'I been there twice, and I'm not a-goin'.' So I'm leaving now and I'm going over to his house and I'm taking him to see a friend of mine, a vascular surgeon, who's going to wait in his office until we get there. He'll examine Mr. Schumer."

I was amazed. It never would have occurred to me to do such a thing. After all, Mr. Schumer had been seen in the ER twice by physicians much more experienced than I was. All I had to go on was my physical exam. Perhaps I'd missed the aneurism the day before. Perhaps it had been there for a long time and the ER docs already knew about it and knew that it wasn't dissecting. What did I know? I'd only been a doctor for a year.

Kathy, however, trusted my physical exam and left for Mr. Schumer's.

She got to his little rose-covered house off a dirt road. She knocked on the door and he answered. He looked awful. She told him he had to go back to the hospital and that she would take him. He told her he didn't want to, didn't need to, and he wasn't going back to the hospital for a third time. He'd seen enough doctors.

Kathy stood outside his house and argued; she wouldn't leave until he got into her car, she told him. So finally he did. Then she drove him to the County Hospital, where her friend the vascular surgeon was doing her a favor and staying late in his office next door. He examined Mr. Schumer and felt the aneurism, which was for sure dissecting because now it was bigger, more than six inches across. So he called for a gurney and took Mr. Schumer over to the hospital for X-rays, and while the X-rays were being done, the aneurism exploded, Mr. Schumer's blood pressure dropped to zero, and he was rushed into the operating room, where Kathy's friend opened the abdomen, clamped the aorta, cut the aneurism out, and then sewed everything up, while Mr. Schumer was getting the five units of blood that make up half the body's blood volume.

By the time I learned from Kathy the next day what had happened, Mr. Schumer was recovering in the ICU. He was still pretty sick, she told me, but would see me for follow-up care as soon as he was discharged.

Ten days later I walked into the examining room and there he was.

Eyes a bit bluer and warmer, smiling, sitting on the examining table, he looked thinner. The first thing he said was that he had a present for me. And out of a brown paper bag he took a glass jar full of a hazy liquid; floating inside it, I saw a large clump of tissue. It was his aneurism. He'd had to fight to get the surgeons to save it for me, he told me, after the pathologists had checked it, and they did, and here it was.

He gave it to me.

I looked at it. I'd never been good at anatomy, that was my friend Rosalind's forte, and it looked like an amorphous mass to me. But what it was, when you think about it, was a life, and I ponder to this day what it meant and what it signified.

It meant that Mr. Schumer's life had been saved by modern technology, by my medical training, by Fast Medicine, but above all, by Kathy, because if Kathy hadn't done what she'd done, no amount of Fast Medicine would have mattered.

So it signified something different. It signified what the real physician must do sometimes to save a life. That I hadn't learned in medical school. No one, not even Dr. Greg, had taught me that. If it had been up to me, Mr. Schumer would have been dead, even though I had made the right diagnosis. Which was, perhaps, why he gave the aneurism to me and not to Kathy. I was the one who needed it.

I did have a good excuse. Two excuses, actually.

First, I wasn't as confident as Kathy was in my perspicacity as a physician. I was barely out of my internship. What did I know? I'd seen an aortic aneurism only once, and Mr. Schumer had been seen twice by experienced ER doctors.

But second, and more important, was that I did not see that my duty as physician was to bully my patient. *Bully* is a tough word, but I'll use it. I'd done what I was supposed to do. I'd followed the Golden Rule, done what I thought I'd want if it were me with that aneurism. I'd diagnosed it and I'd urged Mr. Schumer to go to the ER for a third time. I'd explained what could happen if he didn't go and have it fixed. And he had refused, as was his right, an equal and opposite determination to my own.

But Kathy had recognized what I had not recognized: that Mr. Schumer could not have understood what I told him, because if he had understood, he would have gone to the ER that third time when I'd recommended it. So she did something I never would have thought to do; she took it upon herself to go to his house, in her own car, and insist that he go to the hospital.

Today we've embodied my idea, not Kathy's, in our notions of "informed consent" and "shared decision-making." It's a Fast Medicine approach. It regards human beings as rational, logical—as rational and logical as robots. I, the doctor, inform you, the patient, as to what I've found, what the diagnosis is, and my treatment recommendations, and it's up to you to decide. You can say yes; you can say no. We treat the patient as a rational adult who is literate, educated, and calm, and who has the right to keep his exploding aneurism to himself. Which is fine until you yourself get sick. Then you realize that a sick person, even you yourself, isn't the best person to make decisions for you. Shared decision-making is a fantasy of the healthy.

But Kathy did even more. She knew that another trip to the ER would be as useless as Mr. Schumer thought it would be. Instead she arranged for him to see a vascular surgeon, and put her reputation on the line.

And finally, she made the extra effort.

It was that extra effort that impressed me the most. Getting in her car. Driving way out of her way. Arguing. She took her own time and her own car to do that. I resented the time that medicine took. Even coming home in the evening and reading *Harrison's*, which I did every night, looking up what my patients that day had. I was curious, I was interested, but I also resented the extra effort. Kathy did not resent the time she spent putting straws in people's tracheas or cajoling them into her car. Perhaps it was her upbringing by her grandfather the doctor; perhaps her Seventh-day Adventism; perhaps her sense of a calling. Perhaps it was natural to her, a taste for medicine as natural as her taste for chocolate. For me, medicine was an acquired taste.

And what she taught me that day, and what the aneurism on my desk reminded me of, was that it wasn't enough to diagnose a disease and prescribe the right treatment. That was just being a good doctor. Or even to walk with a patient to the ER. That was just being a better doctor. Kathy showed me that the best doctor diagnoses, prescribes, drives the patient to the ER, and then makes sure he gets the right treatment. By force, if necessary.

Mr. Schumer was a shy man. He had as few dealings with the medical system as he could, but he fought to get that aneurism for me. And I kept it on my desk for a long while, to remind me of what the best doctor, the best nurse, the best person, needs to do, sometimes, to save a life.

NINE

A Slow Medicine Clinic
Before Its Time

After Kathy and that little town of Shafter, I knew I liked medicine, and I put psychiatry behind me. I wasn't yet ready to commit to the three years of an internal medicine residency, however; perhaps I didn't need to. Perhaps I could just be a good clinic doctor and skip that step.

So when my year as locum tenens was up, I moved back to where I'd gone to university, found a clinic with an open doctor position, and drove over for my interview.

It was a pleasant drive. It took me through one of the richest neighborhoods in the state, with impeccably gardened estates and empty streets, then across some railroad tracks, and suddenly I found myself in a little Mexican town hidden away in the suburbs. The main street was lined with shops painted pink, yellow, and blue—*Supertienda, Restaurante, Panadería*—and there was the clinic, with Ms. Jane Lloyd, RN, NP, waiting outside. We went inside and she took me through a waiting room filled with patients sitting on plastic chairs, hands on knees, watching their children play, and then into her office. We sat down and then she turned to me.

Ms. Lloyd was slight and prim, I saw, with pale blue eyes, a small face, and a pinched mouth. Her blond hair was cut in a 1920s bob, and she spoke in a clipped New England accent.

She was looking for a new doctor, she explained, because her general practitioner had just resigned. It was a salaried position—eight-thirty to five, five days a week, and most of the patients were from Mexico. How was my Spanish? Was I comfortable with birth control, venereal disease, and Pap smears? They had a small laboratory—could I use a microscope?

All good, I said. My Spanish was coming along; I could manage a microscope and whatever showed up, as long as there was an emergency room to back me up.

Excellent, she said, and when can you start? Then she smiled. She had a lovely smile that belied her reserve, with just a hint of mischievousness in it. Then we got up and she showed me around.

The clinic was one big space, with a conference table running down its center and six examining rooms against its long walls. Ms. Lloyd opened one of the exam room doors and I peeked inside. Examining table and stool, desk and chair. Simple. Then she took me to the back to see the pharmacy and the supplies.

We were pretty much the pharmacy, she explained, as she opened a cabinet door and showed me jars of pills—antibiotics, blood pressure medicines, anti-inflammatories, steroids. She purchased them from catalogs at pennies the pill so we could give our patients the medications they needed. Here were the pill bottles and here were the labels. Whenever I could, I should prepare my prescriptions myself, counting out the pills, writing the labels, and explaining to the patient how to take them. The receptionist would bill for them.

Next to the pharmacy cabinet was the supply cabinet, with surgical supplies for biopsies, and gynecologic supplies of diaphragms and IUDs.

Orthopedics was here—she opened a closet door and I saw Ace wraps and splints, canes and crutches. Then we walked toward the front, and she told me about the clinic's nurses, Melinda and Becky. They would put my patients in the exam rooms and if I needed help with a procedure, they would assist me. They drew the labs, dressed the wounds, gave the immunizations, went through the mail, and called back patients when necessary. Last, she showed me the "laboratory," which was just a narrow room with microscope, slides, and stains.

Then she walked me through the waiting room to the front door, took my hand in her small and bony one, and shook it.

Ms. Lloyd would turn out to be an excellent administrator. She didn't talk much and she rarely saw patients. She arrived early, left on time, and spent most of the day in her office, and we had no idea what she did in there. No flurry of memos came out of it and she never organized a single staff meeting. Yet we never had an emergency, neither medical nor administrative.

The only crisis we would ever have was during a budget battle in the county when the Board of Supervisors announced it would visit the clinic and take a look at us, and Ms. Lloyd organized it all in a flash. She took photos of our patients and put together a presentation so the supervisors would understand why it was in the county's best interest to continue to fund us. There were photos of the patient crippled by polio thirty years after the Salk vaccine, the patient with active tuberculosis who was a waiter in a popular restaurant. We spoke to them about the contagious parasites we treated in our patients, who were, after all, the child-care workers, gardeners, and elder-care workers of the supervisors' constituency. We never had a problem with the budget after that.

Slowly I began to realize that Ms. Lloyd had a secret to her success. It was her staff, which, though minuscule, was superb, and she put nothing in its way.

For starters there were the nurses, complementary in their tempera-ments, in their strengths and weaknesses. Melinda looked like the girl next door in a 1930s movie. Her hair was long, shiny, and honey-colored, her freckles were fading, and the black eyeliner she wore brought out her green-gray eyes. Lively and enthusiastic, she was inti-mate and warm with the patients, but also careful. She took her job seriously. She knew that at any moment she could make a mistake and someone might die because of it—an insight surprisingly rare in health-care. Becky, on the other hand, was Mexican American, quiet and com-posed. She knew everything there was to know about everyone in town—who was having an affair, who won the lottery, whose grand-mother was sick in Mexico—and somehow, without betraying confi-dences, she managed to convey to us what was really going on with our patients.

The only doctor other than me was Dr. Meryl, the pediatrician. She wore her black hair long, straight, and parted in the middle. Her eyes were wide-set and observant, her voice husky, and her manner brusque. She didn't bother with a white coat but wore polyester slacks, a polyester blouse, and sandals, and she had an unruffledness that was perfect for her tiny patients.

She was also very well trained. She had completed the three years of residency I was avoiding, as well as two years of a fellowship, and every quarter her husband flew her and a group of doctors down to a remote area of Mexico where they provided the only medical care. They would bring the expired medications we could no longer use and old eyeglasses, and there, she told me once, she saw everything. She had a profound expertise underneath that polyester envelope I came to appreciate the day she diagnosed my patient José.

I hadn't known what José had. I walked into the exam room and there he was, sitting on the table with his shirt off. He was thin and small and slumped, with faded brown hair and a furrowed forehead. He came to see me, he told me in Spanish, because for years he'd had no feeling in his hands, and he was a gardener. Did I have any medicine for that?

Then he spread his arms and fingers wide to show me.

His arms were brown and skinny, and both hands looked like claws, with fingers missing. They reminded me of something I'd learned about in medical school but couldn't quite place. So I went out and got Dr. Meryl for a second opinion, and she came in, and José spread his hands for her.

Dr. Meryl stood in front of him with her arms crossed and scanned him slowly, from head to toe and back again. Then she stepped forward and took his right arm in her hands and felt around his elbow, turned his hand over and looked at his palm, dropped it, and did the same on the left. Then she was still. It was the first time I'd ever seen that stillness.

Then she turned to me. "It's leprosy, Victoria."

Leprosy. Wow. I'd never seen a case and I'd thought the disease was pretty much gone.

How was Dr. Meryl so sure it was leprosy?

"Well, see, it's the ulnar nerve hypertrophy here," she said, showing me the lumps at José's elbows. "And the distal wasting here." She showed me his fingers. "The nerves at the elbow enlarge, and that damages the nerves to his fingers, so they get numb and then he burns them or knocks them without realizing it, and the fingers auto-amputate. I've seen it a few times in Mexico."

"Is there anything I can do for him?"

"Well, no, it's too late. You can send him to the leprosy clinic in the City, though, if it's still there. They'll give him dapsone to kill any residual bacteria, but that won't fix his hands, and leprosy's not very contagious, you know."

Then she left.

José didn't seem surprised by his diagnosis. He thanked me, took his referral and left, and that night I took down my books and read about leprosy. The two kinds of leprosy, the lepromatous and the tuberculous, the relationship to armadillos, the lack of acute contagiousness of such a dreaded contagious disease. And then, one week later, Mr. Gonzalez showed up and wanted to know if I had anything for the red patch on his thigh.

I expected to see ringworm—*Tinea corporis*—which was common in our patients and is not a worm but a fungus. But when Mr. Gonzalez hiked up his gown, I was surprised. The red patch had a raised border and it was numb in the center, like the tuberculous leprosy I'd read about the week before. Was that possible? There were only four hundred cases of leprosy in the United States every year. So I went out and found Dr. Meryl and asked her what she thought. Could I have a second case?

Yeah, sure, probably it was leprosy, though I'd have to biopsy it to make sure.

But didn't she think that was strange? To have a second case in one week?

"Not really. In medicine things come in threes. You'll see. You'll have a third case one of these days and then you'll never see it again."

"But why do diseases come in threes? I mean, I can see a second— I've just reviewed leprosy; it's on my mind; I never would have diagnosed Mr. Gonzalez if I hadn't seen José first. But why should I see a third case—and only a third?"

She shrugged. "That's medicine for you. It doesn't make sense, or maybe it makes sense at a deeper level than logic. But keep your eyes open. There's a third case out there for you."

I did biopsy Mr. Gonzalez and it was leprosy, and I sent him, too, to the leprosy clinic. But I didn't see another case. I saw other diseases in series of threes, though, and finally asked a medical transcriptionist about it. Who better would know?

Yes, she told me, the transcriptionists knew about it, too: in medicine a disease comes in threes.

So I kept my eye out. I trusted Dr. Meryl. And finally there it was, years later, lepromatous leprosy in a patient from Peru, and I never expect to see another.

Dr. Meryl's Rule of Threes intrigued me especially because of how she had observed, accepted, and used the irrationality of medicine. After all, it made no sense. Why would you get a run of three patients with the same rare disease, and then no more? If medicine was the science it prided itself on being, that shouldn't be so. You could explain a second case—your mind is attuned, you see it everywhere. But a third, and only a third?

What intrigued me even more was Dr. Meryl. As I watched her scan José and then examine his elbows, she wasn't so much thinking as feeling, performing a quiet, unhurried search inside a huge experience, not linearly but globally, feeling around in her Self for that wholeness, that solution which is the right diagnosis and fits all the clues.

That little clinic kept me on my toes. Its patients could have anything. They would come in with chest pain and it would be leukemia; a lump on the shoulder that would turn out to be sarcoma; a new seizure that would be cysticercosis of the brain. They had every possible parasite, every possible cancer, every possible autoimmune disease. Everything I'd learned in medical school did exist, no matter how rare, and the method I'd been taught—history, physical examination, differential diagnosis—was brilliant. If I followed it step by step, it almost always led me to the right diagnosis, though sometimes the diagnosis it led me to was not what the patient came in for.

So I loved practicing medicine in that little clinic. It was so simple, and its simplicity was its strength. It was just one big room with a table, a few cabinets, some exam rooms, and six people. One receptionist, who combined the roles that would later be apportioned to a community worker, a medical records specialist, a biller, and a patient navigator. Two nurses, who were also the nursing assistants, lab techs, social workers, and caretakers for us physicians. Two doctors, who were, as much as we could be, specialists in infectious disease, endocrinology, genetics, hematology, cardiology, psychiatry, and even a bit of surgery. And Ms. Jane Lloyd, budgeter and jack-of-all-trades. With that we saw more than 7,200 patients a year.

After a few years I began to think I could get away with not doing a residency. Time would tick along, I would see fascinating patients and study medicine on my own. I would never be the doctor that Dr. Meryl was, but the trade-off might be worth it.

And then came our one and only meeting.

It was held in the Doctors' Conference Room of the County Hospital; it was mandatory and all the County doctors attended, in white coats and silk ties, the clinic doctors standing against the walls, the heads of departments sitting at the conference table. At the head of the table were two men in dark suits.

They introduced themselves. They were consultants the county had hired to advise it on what the Health Department could do about its annual budget shortfall of 25 percent, and today they would be presenting their recommendations. The underlying problem, they began, was with the State. In three years it was planning to change how it reimbursed the county for the care of the sick poor from a fee-for-service model, where it paid the county a fee for every service we doctors provided, to a "capitation model," where it would give the county a fixed fee per patient per month, regardless. It was a new model, a way to be cost-effective, and the State predicted it would be 20 percent more efficient than the current model. In a few years, therefore, the county would be getting 20 percent less to run the Health Department, and it had to be prepared.

So what they would be advising was that the county start by giving each doctor a fixed budget, out of which the doctor would pay for his patients' tests, consultations, medications, and hospitalizations. It would be based on current costs, less 20 percent, of course, for the expected efficiency. If we spent less than our budget, we would be eligible for up to a 5 percent bonus; if we spent more, the shortfall would come out of our salary. We would, therefore, have to focus on maintaining our patients' health, since only if our patients stayed healthy would we be able to keep within our budget. But of course, that was the point anyway, wasn't it?

The consultants stopped and looked around the room. Did anyone have any questions?

No one did.

"Well, then, you'll be wanting to get back to your patients, we know. Thanks for being here, and good day."

We all filed out in silence, and as I walked downstairs, I thought about the new plan. It sounded reasonable, in theory, to pay doctors to maintain their patients' health, but in practice my patients didn't have a lot of health for me to maintain. They didn't come to the clinic when they were healthy but when they were sick, and I would therefore have to get them healthy, and how was I going to do that? I had little say in the three determinants of my patients' health: their genetics, their luck, and their choices. The only thing they themselves had control over was their choices, and where did that leave me? I could try to persuade them not to smoke, drink, take drugs, or have unprotected sex; to lose weight, wear their seat belts, take their medications, and get their X-rays, but I did that already and it wasn't particularly successful.

At the bottom of the stairs I ran into my friend Dr. Frack. He was distraught. "Victoria! We'll be responsible for our own budget! If we're over the predetermined amount, it'll come out of our salary!"

I tried to reassure him; I told him I doubted anything would change soon. But the more we talked, the more struck I was by the fundamental contradiction in the consultants' plan. On the one hand, it was based on the idea that doctors were venal, easily incentivized to order too many tests and procedures if that was to our profit, or to order many fewer tests if that was the way the money flowed. On the other hand, the plan relied for its success on the opposite notion, that doctors were ethical and would never *not* order a test if our patient needed it, even if the cost for it came out of our own pocket. It was amazing, when you think about it, how heroic, ethical, saintly! the consultants assumed we doctors are. That contradiction was unconscious and yet crucial to the success of their scheme.

In the county system, the scheme especially did not make sense because we didn't make money on our patients. We received a salary and we already minimized what we ordered because we knew that everything we ordered cost our patients time and money. So we did our own biopsies, consulted specialists over the phone, and tried to prevent hospitalizations by having patients come in every day if they were almost, but not quite, hospitalizable. We already had nothing to gain by ordering things that weren't necessary, and now we would have something to lose if we ordered things that were necessary.

I couldn't imagine trying to practice in such a setup. If I knew that every time I ordered a test it would be coming out of my own paycheck, it would numb my seventh sense.

That meeting decided me. I wouldn't be able to stay at the clinic for long. It was time, therefore, to decide what to do next. I began looking around, going to conferences, seminars, and retreats. Which was how I would meet Mattie and learn there was a way of understanding the body other than the way I knew.

It started with my friend Lee, when she developed asthma.

She'd had asthma as a kid, she told me, but it had gone away and she even smoked, no problem. But now she had started wheezing again and she didn't know what to do. She didn't have health insurance and she made too much money for the clinic.

By then I'd seen a lot of asthma, and since it isn't difficult to treat, I took care of Lee at her home. I started by giving her an inhaler, which helped but only for a bit, so I added theophylline pills. They, too, helped, but pretty soon Lee was wheezing again. Then I added steroids and she improved again but only for a month.

It was frustrating and much more difficult than treating asthma in the hospital or even in the clinic, where the patient comes in suffering, gets better, and leaves. Taking care of Lee at her home let me understand how debilitating the disease is. She missed a lot of work and lost a lot of money, and though she was getting everything I knew to give, her attacks were more and more frequent and severe. Watching them come on was painful. They would start with a coughing fit; Lee would grab and use her inhaler; but despite it, the cough would become spasmodic and then turn into wheezing. When she realized an attack was starting, a look of concentration would appear and her stance would change—hands on hips, hunched over, lips pursed. There would be a controlled panic and a grayness, as she tried to breathe against an implacable restriction.

Finally Lee got so bad she was admitted to the County Hospital. It took the doctors there two days before she improved, and they sent her home with a bag of medicines. Although she was better, her trajectory was worrisome, because the course of adult asthma is downhill. Her wheezing was diminished but not disappeared; it was still there, waiting to clamp down at the first cold, the first whiff of pollen, the first gust of fear or surge of anger. She was not cured but only assuaged.

In the meantime I'd arranged to go on a silent weekend retreat. And after it was over, my assigned roommate and I began to chat. Mattie was lithe, energetic, white-haired and blue-eyed, and she was a healer of the Michio Kushi school, she told me.

What was that? I asked.

It's a version of Chinese medicine, she explained, based on the idea that disease is caused by an imbalance of hot and cold, and wet and dry—yin and yang. Every body has a characteristic healthy balance of the two, and everything we experience—the weather and seasons, our emotions, and what we eat and drink—changes that balance, adding yin and yang in various proportions and so affecting the flow of chi. Chi is our vital force and is supposed to circulate freely through the twelve invisible channels of our bodies. When it gets blocked or depleted, disease arises in the liver, heart, kidneys, spleen, or lungs.

"Asthma?" I asked.

"Yes. Asthma in particular."

"So chi gets blocked in the lungs?"

"No. Asthma is usually a kidney disease. Too much yin, not enough yang; too much cold and wet, not enough hot and dry. The kidney drowns, and, since the liver sends chi to the kidney, when the kidney drowns, the liver's chi backs up into the lungs and causes wheezing. So the treatment of asthma is to balance the excess yin with yang, using yang food and yang herbal medicine."

Lee's swollen face and body, her wet cough, her phlegmatic tone went through my mind. She did look kind of drowned.

"Do you ever make house calls?" I asked.

"I do, but I'm on my way back home to Maryland."

"Stop by before you go. I want you to see a friend of mine."

I had Lee over, and Mattie stopped by on her way to the airport. I introduced them and we all sat down at my dining room table.

Mattie arranged her chair so she was facing Lee. At first she just looked at her. Then she reached out and put her fingers on Lee's wrists and took a pulse for several minutes, first in the right wrist, then in the left. She didn't listen to Lee's lungs but had Lee stick out her tongue and examined it. Then she gave her diagnosis and prescription.

Lee had too much yin and not enough yang, that was why she had asthma. Therefore, she had to increase her yang and decrease her yin. She should start with a strict yang diet for the first ten days—brown rice only. At night she was to eat two umeboshi plums, and three times a day drink four ounces of daikon-radish tea. After ten days, she could begin to liberalize her diet but slowly, with yang foods only, starting with root

vegetables, then fish and chicken. No sugar, fruit, salads, or dairy products. They were too yin. Did we have any questions?

Lee didn't have any questions, but I did. "What should she do about
her asthma in the meantime? It's pretty bad."

"She needs to stop all of her medications immediately. They're
synthetic and that makes them yin."

"All of them? Immediately?"

"Yes."

That was bold. Lee paid for the consultation and we shook hands all
around.

I was amazed to see how quickly Mattie's prescription began to work.
Within forty-eight hours, Lee looked different—not sick. Slimmer, not
so puffy. She held herself taller and moved more quickly, and her
wheezing began to lessen. By day ten, she was well in a way I hadn't seen
in years. Her lungs were clear, her eyes were bright, and her puffiness
had disappeared. It was a cure and I was amazed.

I could understand her cure in two different ways, from two different
points of view.

First, from the point of view of Western medicine, of Fast Medicine.
Mattie had essentially put Lee on a ten-day exclusionary diet, and perhaps Lee had had a food allergy—to milk, for instance. That was not
uncommon. So once Lee stopped eating dairy products, her asthma resolved. The problem with that explanation was that over the succeeding
months, Lee was able to resume eating anything and everything, and
yet her asthma didn't come back.

Or I could take Mattie's point of view, that Lee's asthma was a
symptom of too much yin—too much "cold and wet"—and that rebal-
ancing yin with yang—hot and dry—made her asthma disappear.

That wasn't anything like what I had been taught about the body. But

Lee's cure got me thinking about whether Mattie's point of view might be useful to take now and then, especially for chronic disease and diseases for which modern medicine has no cure.

Because Western medicine, Fast Medicine, I knew by then, did a wonderful job with acute diseases—infections, trauma, catastrophic illness—but not an especially good job with diseases that come on slowly—cancer, diabetes, autoimmune disease. And I liked the idea of having a second model of the body with which to understand my patients. The only thing I didn't like about it was that if everyone had an individual balance of yin and yang, which was what Mattie was implying, then how could we have controlled studies? How could we progress? Which was Western medicine's greatest strength.

But Western medicine had a great weakness, too. It made sense in the details but not as a whole. Although in medical school I had enjoyed learning about the body's machinery—the clotting cascade, the construction of immunoglobulins, the Krebs cycle—in medical practice I'd begun to notice that face-to-face with a patient, the mechanical model of the body did not fit all the evidence. Much of the time, patients got better on their own, and a machine model of the body couldn't account for that. My car never gets over its dead battery or heals the hole in its oil pan.

Perhaps I didn't have to choose. Perhaps I could have two models of the body with which to understand my patients. One model that saw the body as a solid body of miniature factories and broken machines, and a second model that understood it as a body of liquids flowing through channels, of blockages and floods. So I considered. Perhaps what I should do next was learn Mattie's Way—Chinese medicine or Indian medicine, homeopathy or naturopathy.

I thought about Mattie and Lee, and I thought about Dr. Meryl and José.

It was a hinge moment.

Finally I decided—first things first. Before I explored that second medicine, I should finish learning the first. I would bite the bullet. And so I began looking around for a medical residency.

It took me two months to find, but then there it was—the perfect opportunity. "San Francisco Kaiser hospital seeks medical intern to fill unexpectedly vacant residency position."

I called the Dr. Rose listed in the announcement. He took my call right away, and at the end of our chat, was happy to inform me I would be starting my medical internship the second Monday of the next month at seven a.m.

I was not quite as happy as he was, but I was relieved.

TEN

Passing the Point
of No Return

Kaiser hospital in San Francisco, where I would spend the next several years, looked like a 1950s office building. It was a seven-story concrete box with aluminum windows; on the ground floor was a linoleum lobby, with black-and-white photos of retired doctors on its walls, on the top floor was the ICU, and in between were five floors of patient rooms.

Each patient room had four beds, the maximum you could get away with at the time, low ceilings, fluorescent lights, and walls of bilious green. They were not to be confused with hotel rooms; they were not for rest and recovery, but were workmanlike spaces for diagnosis and treatment. They made it clear: the hospital had not been designed by marketeers, nor by idealists, but by businessmen for whom it was a factory for the repair of the sick.

This spareness and economy, this unapologetic budgetarianism, I would later learn, was the hallmark of Kaiser's revolutionary structure, cousin to the HMO model those consultants had been trying to institute at the county. But Kaiser was different from their plan, and better. Created in the 1930s by a socialist-leaning doctor to provide medical care for a monthly fee, it was nonprofit and run by its doctors, who were on salary. There was an overall budget but no specific budget per doctor, and though the attending doctors were conscious of costs, they did not focus on them. They would order whatever the patient needed regardless of cost, once they were convinced it was necessary.

One-quarter of the City's citizenry belonged to the plan, I would discover, and since the hospital had only one hundred medical beds for the 150,000 potentially ill people it served, it was usually 110 percent occupied. This meant there were always ten patients on gurneys in the emergency room, waiting to be admitted. But the patients were working-class, their expectations low, and they were satisfied with the medical care they received even if it was crowded, impersonal, and the doctors were stretched. It was a compromise all around, and, as I would gradually see, it had the strengths of its weaknesses and the weaknesses of its strengths.

For me as intern, however, that year would be exhausting. I was as efficient as I could be, and still I couldn't finish my week's work in less than 116 hours, and there are only 168 hours in a week. Eventually that workload would be outlawed, and I would be glad for the interns who came after, who did not have to work that hard, get so little sleep. I would have been so happy to have had their truncated training. And I would have lost so much, because that internship was an annealing fire.

During that year, I would take care of more than 320 patients, and *Harrison's Principles of Internal Medicine* would come alive, not only because of the breadth of diagnoses I would see but even more because of the minute-to-minute taking care of the patient I would have to do. To admit someone in full-on heart failure and treat him, person-to-person and face-to-face, over the next thirty-six hours, learning what worked and what didn't work, watching him improve! Or sometimes watching him die . . . It would be draining, demoralizing, and I would never want to do it again, but it is what would do the annealing. I would begin to learn the depth of Fast Medicine, I would begin to understand Fast Medicine, cold.

Each patient would teach me something—a trick, an efficiency, a diagnosis. But of all the patients I had that year, it would be Mrs. Irene Carmona who would teach me the most.

It started late one night in February, when I was called down to the emergency room to admit her. She was seventy-three years old and a patient of Dr. Barrows, our blond, blue-eyed, hunky optimist of an oncologist.

For eleven years he'd been treating Mrs. Carmona for chronic lymphocytic leukemia (CLL). It's not the worst kind of cancer to have. Even at the time, it was treatable with an inexpensive oral chemotherapy, chlorambucil. CLL does have a tendency to turn evil eventually, however: to seed the patient's lymph nodes, liver, and spleen with cancer; to cause immunodeficiency and, therefore, unusual infections; and to lead to secondary cancers that pop up in the lung, heart, liver, or brain. But until that night, Mrs. Carmona had been doing pretty well and Dr. Barrows had been proud of her longevity.

She came to the ER because of chest pain, she told me. It had started a few hours before at home, while her husband was watching television and she was working on a jigsaw puzzle. It was a heaviness, worse when she lay down, better when she sat up. No, she didn't have a cough or a fever, though she was, yes, a little short of breath.

She was a remarkably pretty woman, I thought as she talked, especially given her age; she was slim, with mid-length graying brown hair and light-blue eyes, fine-featured and almost stern, until she smiled.

"She turned gray all of a sudden," her husband broke in, "and grabbed her chest and started to choke."

Mr. Carmona was not as handsome as Mrs. Carmona was pretty. He was stolid and square with thinning hair, a slack jaw, small eyes, and his belly hung over his belt.

"I asked her what was going on," he continued. "Did she need water?"

Mrs. C looked over at him. Her eyes were full of anger and spite but she said nothing.

"So I asked her why didn't she take a pain pill? Because last week we were in the emergency room for hours for chest pain, and she's only taken the new medicine for a few days."

"I told him I was going to the hospital whether he took me or not," Mrs. C got out between breaths. Her arms hugged her chest and she was pale.

The possible causes for her chest pain went through my mind. The list was daunting. It could be from her leukemia or a new cancer; it could be from her lungs—pneumonia or a blood clot; or it could be from her heart—angina, a heart attack, or pericarditis, which is an inflammation of the sac around the heart. Her exam, however, was reassuring. I found no lymph nodes and no enlargement of her liver or spleen, which meant it was probably not cancer. Her right lung did have a new effusion—that is, free fluid around it—and her legs were swollen, so perhaps she had a pulmonary embolus, a blood clot to her lungs from her legs. But the test in the ER for that was negative, which left her heart. She did have a murmur, so we admitted her to rule out a heart attack, and over the next several days, with Fast Medicine's oxygen, pain medications, and monitoring, her chest pain resolved, her leg swelling diminished, and she relaxed. She hadn't had a heart attack.

She was just ready for discharge when, on day ten, her heart suddenly went into the regularly irregular rhythm of atrial flutter and she became short of breath and weak. We tried IV medication to get it back into a normal rhythm, and when that didn't work we sent her downstairs to the catheterization lab for cardioversion and an echocardiogram to visualize her heart. The echocardiogram surprised us. It showed idiopathic hypertrophic subaortic stenosis (IHSS), an enlargement of the heart muscle that intermittently can interfere with blood flow. That would explain the symptoms she'd been having of intermittent chest pain and shortness of breath. So we put a tube into her heart to monitor its pressures and transferred her to the ICU for observation.

And that would be the end of that, although we wouldn't know it for a very long time.

Mrs. C would be in the ICU for sixty-three days.

Her husband, with his hangdog face, would come in every day just before lunch. He would sit down in the chair by her bedside, turn on her television, and watch the medical shows, where handsome doctors in crisp white coats stood by beds and spoke to beautiful young patients. When her lunch came, he would eat it. If there were any new get-well cards, he would put them up on the wall so she could see them, and by day 61 of her ICU stay, she had 183 of them. Around two p.m., he would rock himself up out of the chair and lumber out the door.

Mrs. C's two adult children, a lawyer son and a schoolteacher daughter, visited every day. They loved her, they wanted her back. What did she have? they would ask Dr. Barrows, they would ask me. When would she get better? Get out of the ICU? Come home?

Dr. Barrows told them that the reason for their mother's symptoms had most likely been found: it was IHSS with associated intermittent atrial flutter. IHSS explained her chest pain, her shortness of breath, and her frailty. Although there was that new lung effusion on the right. It had been tapped and examined—no cancer, and cultures for infection were also negative—but he had decided, nonetheless, to treat her with a strong antifungal antibiotic, just in case.

But Mrs. C did not improve, despite the antibiotics. She got worse, weaker and frailer, and Dr. Barrows went through the possibilities once again: an immunodeficiency from her leukemia producing an unusual infection; a new cancer; or some other specialty's disease—he would figure it out eventually, he was certain. In the meantime, Mrs. C would stay in the ICU until she stabilized.

But Mrs. C did not stabilize. Every time Dr. Barrows got ready to transfer her out of the ICU, she had chest pain. Or shortness of breath. Or her blood pressure dropped and she had to be resuscitated.

So he kept looking for the diagnosis and had me do every test he could think of—biopsies and bone marrows, blood tests and cultures. But Mrs. C continued to dwindle. She ate less and less and began to lose weight.

As the intern, I saw her every morning and every evening, and if during the day she had chest pain, shortness of breath, an irregular heartbeat, a fever, or a Code Blue, I'd see her then, too; draw her blood, observe her resuscitation, write new orders.

At first she would smile when she saw me.

I would admire her new get-well cards, and as I drew her blood, she would tell me about herself. Frank, her husband, had watched his first wife die of cancer, and when she herself had gotten the diagnosis, he'd been very upset. For a while he even stopped talking to her, but then she took Dr. Barrows's medicine and she didn't die, and eventually he settled with it. But the day she came in, they'd had a fight. He didn't want to take her to the ER, and she'd insisted. There was something wrong with her, she told him, and the doctors didn't know what it was, and their medicine wasn't working. It had been a big fight and she hoped we would find what was wrong. She thought we would—Dr. Barrows was such a good doctor.

But as the weeks went on, she withdrew from me and from everything. She stopped smiling when she saw me and then she stopped talking. She stopped watching television, or greeting her visitors, and stared at the ceiling no matter who was there.

Days and weeks passed and for everything that happened, we had a response. She lost her blood pressure many times, and we found it just as many times. She couldn't breathe, we put a tube down her throat and turned on the respirator. She didn't eat, we fed her with another tube. Her hair fell out, we gave her a little cap.

By month three of Mrs. C's ICU stay, Dr. Barrows had run out of things for me to do. He was convinced it wasn't her leukemia causing her symptoms, and he couldn't find another cancer either. Since it wasn't cancer, she couldn't be dying, and her two children naturally wanted us to keep doing everything. She herself no longer contributed to the discussion.

She was no longer acutely intensive but chronically intensive, however, and so Dr. Barrows demoted her from a single ICU room to a four-bed ICU room. There was not enough wall space in the new room for the get-well cards, and Frank took them down. He still came every day before lunch, though, and her two grown-up children came on alternating days, and I saw her at least twice a day.

But the ICU nurses began to avoid her. They'd liked her. She was an undemanding patient with a gentle manner, and she would get better under their care, the nurses had been sure—everyone did, if they didn't die first. But Mrs. C didn't. She neither died nor got better.

Mrs. C taught me what Fast Medicine could do, what it couldn't do, and what it shouldn't do.

What Fast Medicine could do was keep Mrs. C's body alive almost indefinitely. I could do that in part because I'd taken care of her body so hourly, so minutely, that I could feel when it was about to get sick before it actually got sick. I could tell when she was about to have a fever before she had one, and work up the fever and start antibiotics even before the temperature spike. I could tell when she was about to have chest pain, or go into atrial flutter, or drop her blood pressure before it happened, and I would make the little changes needed to prevent those events.

Plus, I'd developed some Fast Medicine tricks.

For example, I'd learned to use blood to maintain Mrs. C's blood pressure. You're not supposed to do that. You're supposed to use salt-water with sugar and albumin, but that lasts only about twenty-four hours. So when Mrs. C would drop her blood pressure, instead of using water I'd order up blood from the blood bank, which would keep her blood pressure up for days instead of hours.

Of course, my doing all this didn't help Mrs. C, but it did sustain the body of Mrs. C. Which was what the family wanted us to do—everything!—and what Dr. Barrows told me to do, because Mrs. C was not dying.

But that was not what Kathleen would tell me to do.

Kathleen was one of the ICU nurses. She was as young as I was, tall-ish, with gold-red, long, curly hair—yet another nurse named Kathy who would save my life as a physician. There was a reason for all these Kathys, I'd realize much later: the Kathys were Kathys because they were of Irish descent; and the Irish nurses came from an unbroken line of nursing going all the way back to the Middle Ages, when nursing and doctoring were done by nuns and monks as a calling.

It was toward the middle of April when Kathleen pulled me away from Mrs. C's bedside and marched me down the hall of the ICU to the nurses' break room. She sat me down in one chair and herself in another. Then she turned to me and burst out,

"What are you doing! Mrs. C is dying! She's nearly dead! I don't know why, you don't know why, but she's never going to leave this ICU, not ever!"

Then she sat back and looked at me.

I didn't know how to respond. "Well, I know it seems hopeless and probably is, but Barrows says she doesn't have cancer but some infec-tion or autoimmune disease and once we find it we can treat it and then she'll get better and go home. And until we do, we support her in the ICU as long as necessary."

Kathleen shook her head. "Look at her! She has no more IV sites, her skin is disintegrating, her teeth have fallen out! She is never ever again going to hold her granddaughter on her lap, she's not ever going out of here, not on her own two feet, not in a wheelchair, not on a gurney. She's past the point of no return."

No one had ever told me about that in medical school, about a point of no return. It was the first I'd heard of it. It wasn't something that Fast Medicine acknowledged, that there was a point of decay, disease, deterioration, after which the body cannot recover. "A downward spiral," as my soon-to-be executive director would call it, with his ironic Texan twang, when the cells of the body can no longer maintain their structure, their complexity, their unity. Of course, you can have a burn or an accident from which you can't recover—everybody knows that. But that some process—an infection, a cancer, despair, loneliness, anger—could go on too long for the body to recoup. . . . I hadn't realized that such a point existed, and Mrs. C had gone on so long that I hadn't noticed—the aging face of your once overwhelmingly loved lover—that she had reached it.

So I got up and went into Mrs. C's room, stood by her bed, and looked. And saw.

That was another distinction Fast Medicine didn't pay attention to. Looking and seeing. I'd been at Mrs. C's Code Blues, taken blood from her ever-more-fragile veins, checked her labs twice a day, but I hadn't *seen* her for a very long time.

Now I did see, and I was shocked. She lay on her back unmoving, while her eyes roved across the ceiling. Her arms outside the covers were swollen and boggy. Her hair was gone, her face yellowish, her lips black, her teeth broken. She looked like a death mask.

Kathleen was right. Mrs. C had passed the point of no return. She was dying and it didn't matter what she was dying of—whether an infection, a cancer, or something we hadn't yet diagnosed. She was never going to get better, and what *were* we doing?

Not only had I not looked and seen Mrs. Carmona for a long time, but neither had Dr. Barrows. He was intent, focused; she would not die of his disease, which was cancer. But we shouldn't be doing what we were doing, and I needed to say something about that to Dr. Barrows, I decided. Get him to notice, as Kathleen had done for me.

But how?

It was tricky. I was an intern and a woman, so twice invisible. Dr. Barrows had never said a word to me, except for orders, though we'd been taking care of Mrs. C together for fifty-six days. Still, I could try.

So the next morning when he came by on rounds, I asked him what were we doing? Mrs. C was dying.

"No, she's not," he replied. "Her cancer is gone. She has a fungal infection, most likely. And if we can get rid of it, she has a good chance of leaving here."

"Can't we talk to her husband? Her kids?"

He looked at me coldly. "She's not dying."

I did have one chance. But I didn't take it.

It came a week after Kathleen took me into the break room.

Mrs. C had once again developed a cough and I was sure it was because she was in heart failure, with fluid backing up into her lungs. She needed, therefore, to be dried out. Since Dr. Posen, the cardiologist, was coming by for morning rounds, I made sure to be at her bedside when he arrived with his residents so I could hear his diagnosis. They all gathered around and Dr. Posen picked up the nursing clipboard to see the Swann-Ganz (SG) values of pressures in her heart.

Her SG was 5, he noted to the group.

In the usual patient, an SG of 5 means that the patient is dehydrated and needs fluids, and Dr. Posen told me to order two liters of fluid for Mrs. C.

But in Mrs. C's case, I knew that this wasn't right. I knew her body well, and she was so frail that for her an SG of 5 most likely meant the opposite, that she was fluid-overloaded—drowning—and should be diuresed, dried out.

"But what do you think about her albumin?" I asked him. "It's only 0.7. Couldn't that change how we interpret her SG? She has a cough. Couldn't she be fluid-overloaded and not dehydrated, and still have an SG of five?"

"No," he answered, and went on with his group to the next patient.

But I knew, I just knew, that Mrs. C needed the opposite of what Dr. Posen had ordered. If I did give her those two liters of fluid, she would drown, code, and perhaps die.

What should I do?

There were two opposing ethics—two ways to be right and two ways to be wrong. One ethic was to do what was best for Mrs. C, which was to give the fluids Dr. Posen had ordered and let her go. But that would mean consciously doing what I believed was medically wrong. It would mean not being the best doctor I could be, and that was a value I held dearly. A perhaps selfish value. I think the truly brave person, the most enlightened person, would have followed Dr. Posen's orders, given the fluids, and allowed Mrs. C to die.

I remembered the beginning of the Bhagavad Gita, when Prince Arjuna asks Krishna whether it is ethical for him, the Prince, to join the battle of one side of his family against the other. Krishna answers, "If any man thinks he slays and if another thinks he is slain, neither knows the ways of Truth. The Eternal in Man cannot kill; the Eternal in Man cannot die, wherefore, do thy duty."

But what was my duty? Was it to do what was best for Mrs. C? Or what was best for Mrs. C's body?

To this day I am not happy about my decision.

I was pretty sure that an X-ray of her lungs would show that Mrs. C was not dehydrated but fluid-overloaded, and I was also pretty sure that trying to get Dr. Posen to look at that X-ray and change his decision would be awkward and probably useless. But later that morning

Dr. Fong was coming by. He was big, smart, and warm, and his was an open mind. So I ordered a chest X-ray, put it up by Mrs. C's bed, and was at her bedside when he came around.

I asked him to look at the X-ray with me.

"Hmm. Yes. Obviously she's in heart failure. Fluid overload."

"So she doesn't need fluid?" I asked him.

He looked at me strangely. "Of course not."

"Dr. Posen ordered two liters of fluid this morning because her SG pressure was five. Could you talk to him?"

A little smile appeared on Dr. Fong's face. "Sure. I'll talk to him."

Thus Mrs. C did not get those two liters of fluid and did not die that day or the next. Instead she struggled and dwindled and fought and faded, and looked like a skeleton on the day she did die, which was at ten a.m. on Sunday, May 1, the sixty-third day of her ICU stay, two hours after I went off service and handed her over to my fellow intern, the blithe Dr. Sturgeon. I didn't explain to him about her worsening cough, her need for a blood transfusion if her pressure dropped—all my tricks—and he didn't ask. Dr. Sturgeon was a realist and never split hairs.

And why did she die just when she did, exactly two hours after I went off service?

I wasn't there, so I can't say for sure. But I wasn't there, and that probably had something to do with it. They say, and I've seen, how people somehow keep themselves alive until a graduation or a wedding, until some loved or hated person arrives or departs. So perhaps it wasn't so much, or only, my assiduous tweaking of all Mrs. C's labs and numbers that kept her alive so long. Perhaps it was my presence, my attention, my witting care.

And so, with Mrs. C's death my annealing internship came to a close.

Because of her, I'd learned what Fast Medicine couldn't do, which is fix someone if something is In the Way of that person getting better.

It can be anything—physiological, environmental, psychiatric, mental, or spiritual; bacteria, fluid in the lungs, home life, drugs, alcohol. And unless what is In the Way is identified and removed, it is not possible for someone to heal. We never found out what was In Mrs. C's Way.

From Mrs. C, too, I'd learned what I shouldn't do with Fast Medicine. I should never again be in a position where I had to keep someone in her situation alive. I had to keep a global view of my patient in front of me, and if necessary tell the family and the patient what Kathleen told me—Alas, you're not going to get well; you're going to die. You've passed the point of no return. We don't know why, but it would be wrong to keep going.

Even though one true tenet of medicine is not to take hope away.

And if the family, or even the patient, insists—Do everything—when the case is hopeless, it is not a choice for me to give or them to make. "Patient autonomy" goes only so far. No patient, no family, can know what they are saying when they say, Do everything. Being a doctor means seeing things clearly, explaining things clearly, but in the end, if necessary, it means saying no.

That's not to say that having a living will or Advanced Life Directives isn't a good thing. It was helpful to hear "Everything!" from Mrs. C's family. It gave us a sense of where she fell on the spectrum from "do nothing" to "do everything." But applying those wishes and ideas in a practical situation means choosing medical interventions, and that cannot be done in advance. When you get really sick, following your directives becomes a moving target and a judgment call. What is a reasonable "Everything!" today is not the same "Everything!" tomorrow. What happened with Mrs. C was that we did not apply the perspective Kathleen gave me to her family's "Everything!" We should have understood that meant "Everything that is helpful—at this point." And judged when that was a point of no return.

Finally, from Mrs. C I learned what I could do with Fast Medicine, which was keep a body alive for a very long time. And though my doing so had done Mrs. C no good—it had done her harm—it left me forever after with a certain kind of confidence. It was the confidence the best attendings had, almost a tuning fork for the body.

Confidence, from the Latin, *confidere*: to trust, to have faith in. From Mrs. Carmona I had learned to have faith in the body, but not exactly the body as a machine or a collection of machines. Her body did obey the laws of the body I'd been taught, but in an individual, connected, and harmonious way, and over those months I had learned to know that way with my own body. I knew just how, as her blood count would fall, ever so slightly, her heart would speed up, ever so slightly, and then because of her IHSS and low albumin level, fluid would back up into the lungs, and she would get, again, ever so slightly, restless. I would feel that restlessness, that sense of unease, disharmony, in my own body, and I would correct, almost unconsciously, whatever it was that was off.

It was subtle, but there was some global way I was registering her state of health and illness, not the individual changes but the whole change. Just as a musician registers the harmony of a piece of a music, my body, my self, had somehow learned to tune itself to hers. And if I could do that with one patient, then I could do that—whatever it was I was doing—with others.

In Which Fast Medicine and Slow Medicine Come Together

My internship year was now over, but I didn't directly begin the next two years as a medical resident. Dr. Rose had to rearrange the schedule for me to do so, and that was going to take him a year. The upshot was that now I had twelve months away from the hospital to rest, study, and have adventures. I'd heard it was possible to walk across Nepal to Mount Everest, and I decided to do that.

What intrigued me about Nepal was how medieval it was supposed to be. I'd been intrigued by the Middle Ages my whole life—by its castles and cathedrals, its bells tolling and market people calling out their wares. By its values—fighting dragons, rescuing damsels, being honest, faithful, and true. By its culture, which focused on a life beyond the material—hermits in their chapels, monks in their monasteries, pilgrims on the road. The Middle Ages knew that Judgment Day would come, and with it, retribution. In the end there would be justice, and life would make sense.

I'd always wondered what it must have been like, really, and Nepal seemed about as medieval as you could get. Except for in the capital of

Kathmandu, it had no telephones, no cars, and no roads, and the only way to get someplace was to walk there.

So I found a trekking group, signed up as its physician, and we walked across the country from its southern border with India to its northern border with Tibet. It was fascinating. We walked from valley to valley over high passes, and saw how the physiognomy of the people gradually changed from Indian to Tibetan, how the religion gradually changed from Hindu to animism and Buddhism, how the crops and countryside changed.

But the medicine did not change, and I was most surprised by what we did not encounter—no medicine at all, neither Fast nor Slow. I hadn't imagined our Middle Ages to be as medically bereft as Nepal seemed to be. Not only did we find no doctors, hospitals, or clinics, but there didn't seem to be the simplest medical knowledge, not even of hygiene. Babies were placed outside while their mothers worked in the rice fields, and their noses and eyes ran and were covered with flies. In the rivers, boulders were used as latrines, even while downstream, water was being taken for cooking and drinking. In the houses, there were no fireplaces or chimneys; women cooked over an open fire with just a hole in the roof for smoke to escape. So the most common ailment was red eyes, and the most common childhood injury, burns.

As we walked I saw infections, disfigurements, leprosy, and I wondered if that was how our Middle Ages had been. It was hard to believe. It was medieval Europeans, after all, who built the cathedrals and developed our law, libraries, and universities. There must have been some kind of medical knowledge. Nepal itself was not unsophisticated, and perhaps its medicine was around me somewhere, but I sure couldn't find it.

As the trek physician I was lucky. Everyone stayed healthy. But I did get to be a doctor once. It was during the second week when we were, therefore, an eight-day journey from civilization.

We were walking from one high pass to another on a path that went along the side of a mountain which was terraced with rice paddies. Our caravan was spread out in a long line. First Suresh, our Nepalese leader; then the porters with our tents, provisions, and my medical trunk; then our American leader and the four of us tourists on the trip. I was at the very end. I had just made it to the top of the next rise when I saw down below a man coming out of a little wooden house set back from the rice paddies. He waited until the caravan got to him, then stopped Suresh and talked to him. Suresh gestured up to me and continued past. The man waited on the path until I got down to him. He was wearing khaki shorts, tall and thin, with a high forehead, deep-set eyes, and a mustache drooping over a Hapsburg chin.

"Are you the doctor?" he said, in a refined English accent.

"Yes, I'm the doctor."

"Could I ask your help? Seems I've a splinter in the back of my knee. Had it for a few days, can't seem to get to it myself."

"What have you tried?" I asked, imagining the poking, the knife, the infection.

"Oh, I sterilized a needle, you know, with a match, tried for a bit, but just can't get to it, back of the knee, you see. Now, it's, well—a bit warm, red, starting to hurt."

We both knew where we were, in the middle of the Middle Ages, with distance measured in footsteps, not miles, in days, not minutes. In the entire country, there was not a single helicopter, and the only place for a plane to land was a day's walk away. With no hospital or clinic near, no possibility of IVs or nursing care, an infection could be fatal.

"Sure, I'll take a look."

He turned around and started to hike up his shorts.

"Not here. Let's go into my 'office.'"

"Yes. Right. Much better."

I followed him into his little house, which was made of wood, airy and clean. There was a sofa by the window, a coffee table, and a tiny kitchen, where I washed my hands.

The medical trunk was already down the hill but I carried an aluminum tin in which I had everything I might need for a simple emergency. Mr. English put a blanket and a clean sheet on the floor between the sofa and the coffee table, and then lay facedown so I could get a good look.

It was easy. A thick wooden splinter was embedded right above the back of his knee, and the area around it was swollen, red, and hot. It was infected and he could never have gotten that splinter out himself.

I took out what I'd need from my kit and laid it on the table—iodine swabs, sterile needle, scalpel, mosquito clamp. I cleaned off the skin, uncovered the splinter with the needle, and used the clamp to grab it. I pulled and it slid right out. It wasn't a splinter after all but a large thorn, and it came out whole, no dirt or debris left behind. Then I applied antibacterial ointment and covered it with a Band-Aid.

Mr. English stood up and straightened his clothes. I made him a packet of antibiotics and then put my things away. He'd had a tetanus shot before coming out there, he told me, and I had him swallow the first two antibiotic pills in front of me. Then he walked me out of his little house and we stood together, mountains surrounding us, and looked for my caravan, which was now all the way down the hill. He shook my hand, thanked me, told me he had recently retired as Chief Magistrate of Hong Kong, and would I like a cup of tea?

"No, thanks. I should catch up to my group. But remember—two pills, three times a day, and keep the wound clean."

"Of course."

I took off and he watched until I was down the hill and caught up to my group.

I was sure he would follow my instructions, and that his wound would heal without incident. What struck me, though, as I walked, was what a simple thing it had been—a thorn in an inaccessible place—and yet how potentially devastating. It hadn't needed a doctor but it had needed another person, soap and water, a sharp needle, and a shiny stainless-steel instrument of German manufacture, which could snap onto that thorn and pull it out whole, and there was nothing like it in all of Nepal. The only tools we'd seen were *kukris*, homemade knives the men carried. We'd passed the workers digging iron out of the ground, the smelting shacks where the iron became primitive steel, and the blacksmiths hammering out the knives. The men used them for everything, from cutting down a tree to picking their teeth, but no *kukri* could have gotten out that thorn.

Had our group not come along with Fast Medicine in a little tin, Mr. English's thorn might well have festered and turned septic, the skin around it getting redder, hotter, and more painful. His body might eventually have ejected the thorn on its own, but just as likely the infection would have spread up his thigh into his groin, and thence into his bloodstream. He would have gotten a fever, taken to his bed, become delirious, lost his blood pressure, and died. He was, after all, eight days from a hospital. In the Middle Ages, people often died of such little things—rich, powerful people. Richard the Lionheart died of infection from an arrow to his shoulder; the Holy Roman Emperor Frederick II of diarrhea.

So Mr. English put the Middle Ages into perspective for me. Whatever I missed from them—their quiet, their values, their worldview—I was glad of my Fast Medicine technology: morphine and iodine and my beautiful steel instruments, sterile-packaged needles, and antibiotics. Mr. English marked the beginning of a change of heart. If Mrs. Carmona's tragic dying was an example of too much Fast Medicine, then the mosquito clamp in my aluminum tin was an example of just the right amount of Fast Medicine for the job.

I had to earn a living during that intermission year, so I signed up with a locum tenens agency, where I would substitute for doctors taking their vacations. I would walk into a medical practice in a city, suburb, or village and see the many ways medicine could be done—the elegance or shabbiness of the office, the power or lack of power of the nurse, the different ways different doctors thought about their patients, the medications they used, their styles.

Some doctors treated everything all the time, I learned, while others hardly treated anything at all. Some doctors worked up every symptom and used Fast Medicine to the max, others led with tincture of time. Some were authoritative and brisk, others skeptical and humorous, a few kindly and even bumbling. But every style worked pretty well, because over time a doctor collected the patients he deserved—the conservative wait-and-see doctor collected conservative wait-and-see patients; the aggressive, active doctor collected patients who liked getting tests and taking pills. So when I replaced Dr. Y, all I had to do was figure out his style and not get in its way.

After two months of doing locums I found a practice that suited my style. It was a rural clinic on a bluff overlooking the ocean and provided the only medical care for hundreds of miles around. Its staff was tiny—a receptionist and another Nurse Kathy with the common sense you needed for the job. Its patients were mainly middle- and working-class, but there were also the rich of a nearby second-house enclave and a tribe of Native Americans on a reservation. The deal was that I would be the doctor for the clinic every other month until my residency started up again. I would be on call every fourth night and every fourth weekend, and if someone had to be seen off-hours, I would take care of the patient by myself at the clinic.

During the day, with the staff around and light in the sky, being on call wasn't too stressful, but it sure was at night. I was the only doctor for several hundred square miles and the nearest hospital was a two-hour drive away. Anything could happen, and it did: a laceration to sew up, a gastrointestinal upset, a drunken man with a prostatic obstruction to treat and I'd never done that before. If it hadn't been for that internship, I never would have been able to do it, but it had prepared me to be in such a role, which was alone. The operator would page me and I would answer the call; I would meet the patient at the clinic, unlock the door, put a chart together, listen, diagnose, and treat; then I would clean up, write the bill, and, strangest of all, take money for my services.

I had one big moment. It began the afternoon of Memorial Day.

I was sitting cross-legged with my shoes off at the dining room table, reading *Harrison's*, when the phone rang. It was the answering service putting a patient's wife through. I began to put on my shoes. That's one of the things I'd learned to do that year. The natural instinct is to try to dissolve worry over the phone, to find a reason not to have to leave home and go out into the cold, adversarial universe. But this instinct leads to mistakes, I'd discovered, to misjudgments. So I put my shoes on when I took a call. That way I'd have to be convinced *not* to go.

"I'm so sorry to bother you at home, Doctor, but my husband's doctor told me to call if his pulse ever got below forty-five."

"Why were you taking your husband's pulse?" I asked.

"Oh, I always do. I'm supposed to, before I give him his medication."

Ahhh. I knew the medication well. It's a blood pressure medicine, and it always slows the pulse. That is, in part, its point. So it was probably nothing serious, and I stopped putting on my shoes.

"Well, what does it usually run?"

"Oh, fifty or fifty-five."

"What did you get today?"

"Forty-two."

A normal pulse rate is above 60. Most people can manage with a pulse above 50, but at 42 there's not enough blood circulating to the brain and a patient can get confused, fall, or even have a seizure. Plus, I didn't know what was causing such a drop. The medication he was taking shouldn't drop the pulse that low. I tied my shoes.

"Did you give him his medicine anyway?"

"No."

"That's good. That's very good. . . . Sounds like I need to see him, though. Can you bring him into the clinic?"

"Now? It's Memorial Day."

"I'm afraid so. I need to at least take his pulse and get his blood pressure myself."

"Won't tomorrow be soon enough? I know he won't want to go."

I put on my sweater.

"Better to come in now, to be sure. I'll meet you there."

It wasn't a long drive, and I got to the clinic before they did.

I unlocked the doors, turned on the lights, and went into our ER, which was simply an examining table in a large room. I put on my white coat, pulled a fresh tissue cover over the table, opened the storage cabinet, and took out an IV bag, plastic tubing, and needles. I didn't think I'd need them. Probably it was his medication that was causing the slowed pulse. But you never know, and I'd learned to be a bit of a nurse in my months there.

Mrs. Sturm arrived in a white Cadillac with Mr. Sturm in tow. She was dressed for the doctor's in suit, stockings, and lipstick, and Mr. Sturm was in slacks, open shirt, and sports coat. I don't know how she'd managed that, because Mr. Sturm was not all there. He was slow, stiff, and confused even about where to put his feet.

I sat down next to him in the waiting room and took his pulse. It was 36, and this was not good. This I couldn't handle. Mrs. Sturm had been right. The pulse she'd taken a few hours before must indeed have been 42 and now it was 36 and Mr. Sturm was confused. Perhaps he'd had a right-sided heart attack that knocked out his sinus node, the small collection of specialized cells which sends a jolt of electricity every second through the heart muscle and causes it to beat. The heart does have a backup—a second group of cells that can take over if the sinus node fails—but it beats much more slowly, in the thirties. Or perhaps his atrial-ventricular node was blocked. Its job is to regulate the pace of beats from the sinus node, and if it is damaged it can slow the pulse down too much. Or perhaps Mr. Sturm had sick sinus syndrome, where the sinus node as it ages begins to speed up and slow down irregularly. In any case, there was no way I could take care of him alone in the clinic on the bluff. He needed a hospital—fast, before his pulse went down further and he died.

I needed help.

I led Mr. Sturm into our ER and had him lie down on the table, and while I was putting together the IV, I called Andy, who was the owner of the general store down the road. He was the closest person, and he also happened to be a volunteer fireman, he told me on the phone. He came right over.

"You've got two choices, Doc, if he needs to go to the hospital and be monitored along the way."

"Put on the oxygen, will you, Andy?"

"Sure . . . You can call the paramedics from Santa Rosa. They'll come out in their ambulance but it'll take a couple of hours both ways. Or you can get the helicopter."

"Help me get this coat off, will you? . . . There's a helicopter?"

"Yeah, but you have to go with him. There's a pilot and a copilot but no one has medical training."

I got the IV started. Thank God. And it was running. Miracle! I had access. "Okay, let's call the helicopter. He can't wait four hours."

So Andy called, and while we waited for the helicopter I got an EKG on Mr. Sturm. Thank God also for all those horrible nights as an intern: I got it and I read it, and, sure enough, it looked like a slow ventricular rhythm down to 32 by this time. I went out to the waiting room, sat down, and explained what was going on to Mrs. Sturm. We were going to helicopter her husband to the County Hospital, and she should meet us there. We would do everything we could, but it was very serious.

She appeared composed and attentive, though there was the slightest stiffening of her shoulders, settling of her face. She would wait until we left, she said, and drive herself to the hospital.

Then we heard the helicopter and I went outside. It descended from the sky and landed on the bluff in its strange, insectoid way.

Andy and I went over to meet the pilots, and then we went back into the clinic, helped Mr. Sturm off the table, and switched his oxygen to the helicopter's oxygen. We couldn't take the IV bag because there was no place to hang it in the helicopter, so I put in a heplock, which is a tube that keeps the vein open and can be used to inject drugs. Andy and I managed to get Mr. Sturm into the backseat of the helicopter, and then, with the copter's propeller turning, I went around to the left and ducked in next to him. Andy would lock up the clinic.

It was very noisy inside and the copilot handed me headphones. That's how we would communicate, he gestured. Last, he passed me a bag of medications.

With the roof of the helicopter curving over our heads and down behind our backs, it felt just like being in the backseat of an old Volkswagen. There was the rounded windshield in front and the cramped seat, and I was sitting right up against Mr. Sturm, who was incommunicado, although his eyes were still open and he was upright. Then, just like in a VW, the pilot pushed the throttle forward and there was a lurch, but instead of going forward, we went straight up. And up. Soon we were high in the sky—higher than the coastal mountains and flying toward them. Then the copilot turned around and handed me a pulse monitor, and I attached it to Mr. Sturm's left forefinger. His pulse was down to 30.

I took his hand to check the pulse myself. His hand was cold and floppy, and his pulse was not only slow but weak. Then he lost consciousness and his head slumped against my shoulder.

"Do you guys have atropine?" I asked through the headphone mic. Atropine can speed up the heart, although you never know for sure what a medication is going to do.

"I don't know. Look in the bag."

I opened the brown cloth bag they'd given me. It was filled with medications, and yes, there were two ampules of atropine in premedicated syringes.

We were flying over the mountains now, and Mr. Sturm's pulse was down to 28. I was reluctant to give the atropine to a patient I didn't know well, in the cramped back of the helicopter, because if something unexpected occurred—if it stopped his heart, for instance—I would have no room to resuscitate him. Or if, on the other hand, the atropine, which also has brain effects, caused agitation, it could be a mess in that little space, given the needle, the oxygen, and the thin walls of the helicopter. Should the pulse get down to 22, I decided, I would give the atropine, regardless. Mr. Sturm was getting colder and colder and I so didn't want him to die on me. When his pulse got down to 23, I took a deep breath and let it slowly out, prepared the atropine, and injected it.

I counted to ten as the medication circulated. And then, miraculously, Mr. Sturm's pulse began to rise: 25, 30, 36, 42. At 45 he began to stir. At 48 he raised his head off my shoulder and his hand warmed up.

By this time, we were over the mountains and starting to descend to the helicopter pad on the roof of the County Hospital. Mr. Sturm's pulse was up to 50 and we landed. People rushed toward us, nurses and doctors with oxygen, IV poles, medications, and a gurney. I was never so glad.

I got out of the helicopter and made my report. Mr. Sturm was put on the gurney and trundled off to the ICU, and then the pilots asked, "Shall we take you home?"

The flight back was spectacular. We flew over the mountains and then up the coast along the edge of the water. The fog had cleared and the Pacific, the peaceful ocean of California, spread out north and south and west. There was the green coast on the right and the white waves on the left that marked the end of civilization, and then we were back at the clinic. We landed on the bluff. I thanked the pilots, they took off, and I reopened the clinic to clean up.

The next morning, my nurse Kathy arrived.

"Heard you had an exciting day yesterday," she said.

"How did you know about that?"

"Oh, everyone knew about that. . . . How did you like the helicopter ride?"

"It was great," I said. "Amazing . . . I'd never been in a helicopter before."

"You liked it?"

"Yeah."

"Well, just to let you know. That's our third helicopter."

I missed a beat.

"What happened to the other two?"

Kathy had an amused smile in her eyes as she scrutinized my own. "The other two crashed. The first one killed the pilots and our doctor. That's why we don't have a permanent doctor. And the second one just killed the pilots."

I would so love to tell you how well Mr. Sturm did, how he survived and came home to his wife and his blood pressure medicine, his sports coat and his evolving dementia. But he didn't, although he didn't die right away. He lingered in the hospital for two months and then he died.

So maybe it would have been better if I hadn't used the atropine, called the helicopter, met him in the clinic, or put on my shoes. I have no way of knowing. Maybe those extra two months were a good thing—time to say good-bye, to tie up loose ends. Though I doubt it. Those are the months in which, health-care economists tell us, almost all the expenses of our health-care system occur, and I believe them. Most likely it was suffering I brought to Mr. Sturm and Mrs. Sturm and his family. I thought of Mrs. Carmona, and the flogging of the dead and the dying. But that is not why I remember this story or what happened for me in it.

It was the moment I made the decision to give the atropine. Alone in the back of the helicopter with a person dying next to me. It was the only decision to make, but whatever happened—and I didn't know what would happen—would be my responsibility. I didn't have all the information; it would be easy afterward to second-guess myself, or for someone else to second-guess me. But that would be later, and this was now.

It was the accepting of that responsibility, by myself, in the sky. Searching through the bag with the shaking of the helicopter and its noise, and taking it on. It was the moment when the flowing rock cools and sets, anneals, hardens and crystalizes, all the atoms in place.

After that, I knew myself as a doctor.

What do I mean?

There's a lot more to being a doctor than the accepting of responsibility, but it starts there. This is what is so detrimental about algorithms, regulations, requirements, and mandates. They lift that mantle of responsibility off the doctor and turn him or her into a provider, a middleman, someone who takes the box of healthcare off the truck and delivers it. He can always point to someone or something else—she made me do it; it made me do it—Adam in the Garden of Good and Evil, pointing to Eve—she made me do it; and Eve pointing to the serpent; he made me do it.

It is the taking of responsibility that marks the distinction between apprentice and journeyman. Before you accept it, you're an amateur, a student, an intern—provisional. There's always someone else to ask, to pass the key decision to. But in the helicopter, there was only me. I had the duty and the obligation; and I had the knowledge and experience. I wasn't certain I was right. But I was certain it was the only thing to do, and that I could manage whatever happened in consequence. By the time we landed, I knew that something had changed for me, forever.

And so intermission came to a close.

During it I had learned what a world would be like without Fast Medicine—without its logic, method, and technology—and I appreciated Fast Medicine all the more. I had been shaken by Mrs. Carmona, and by the experience as an intern of seeing many successful treatments of deadly diseases but no cures. The pneumonia case went home coughing with his treated pneumonia, though not dead, to be sure; the cancerous with her treated cancer, and all the side effects of that, but not cured, merely suffering prolonged, I had thought. In Nepal I learned I'd been selling Fast Medicine short, and my attitude toward it changed.

From all those locums, I learned a Slow Medicine lesson: how individual medicine was. It wasn't true that one size fits all, that everyone or no one should have that treatment or this pill. Rather, the right answer had to do with style, with who you were, who the patient was. Later, when I studied medical history, I would discover that Hippocrates had already known that: It doesn't matter so much, he wrote, which disease the patient has, but rather, which patient has the disease. Now I would add, and which doctor has the patient!

The third lesson I learned that year was neither a Slow Medicine nor a Fast Medicine lesson, but a medicine lesson. That taking of responsibility, which the surgeon does every time he or she picks up a scalpel, and physicians do every time they pick up a pen, and pathologists do every time they screw down their magnifying lens on a specimen and pronounce it as "cancer," or not.

And now, with my Intermission year over, I would go back to the hospital and the City and find myself, unexpectedly, in the eye of the eye of a storm.

ELEVEN

Turnaround

The storm was AIDS, although that wasn't its first name. Its first name was GRID—gay-related immune deficiency—so named because gay men had started showing up in Los Angeles, New York, and San Francisco with bizarre infections and rare cancers that could only be due to an immune-system dysfunction. I'd read the first reports while I was still at Jane Lloyd's clinic, and shortly after, a young gay man presented with a telltale symptom, lymphadenopathy—enlarged lymph nodes all over his body. He was my first case, and I sent him up to San Francisco for a workup.

By the time I was an intern, we were beginning to see a few cases—frightening, fatal cases we did not know how to manage. We followed the Fast Medicine script that had been so successful with other diseases, working up the chief complaint—the main symptom—methodically. So a patient who came in with a cough and fever got a workup for pneumonia; with a headache and fever, a workup for meningitis; with chest pain and fever, a workup for endocarditis. Those first few patients weren't put in isolation, however, and we didn't even wear gloves, and as we worked them up they would deteriorate into a mass of flesh with tubes within a week.

Something new was going on. Something we hadn't seen before. What was it, and what was its cause?

There were two distinct hypotheses. It was a time of sexual experimentation, another aspect of that Aquarian Revolution, as well as drug experimentation, and there had been a predictable increase both in sexually transmitted diseases—syphilis, gonorrhea, herpes—and also in overdoses and skin infections from needle use. The two hypothetical causes of GRID corresponded: the first hypothesis was that it was a sexually transmitted viral infection causing immunosuppression, and the second that it was a cumulative injury to the immune system from recreational drugs and anonymous sex.

So you could say there was a hypothesis of the Left and a hypothesis of the Right, and Fast Medicine chose the first. It was impressive to watch the scientific method in action, though not exactly clean. That is to say, once Fast Medicine chose its hypothesis—that GRID, renamed AIDS once cases started appearing in heterosexuals, was caused by a viral infection and was therefore identifiable with its tools—its search was objective, but it ignored any evidence that didn't fit its hypothesis.

We who were seeing the disease, however, were sure it was infectious. Dr. Dobbins, one of our ER docs, had even identified its acute phase, he told me one night—a fine pink rash. He was a year ahead of everyone else, but who except an ER doctor in the heart of San Francisco could have observed the acute phase of this new disease?

During my intermission year, scientists began intensely researching, trying to figure out whether it was a known or unknown infection, and they discovered a new virus they named "human immunodeficiency virus"—HIV.

Since meanwhile the 24/7 partying in the Castro was continuing, by the time I got back to the hospital, those few first patients had turned into a storm. The arithmetic was frightening: 25 percent of San Francisco belonged to Kaiser, and of that 25 percent, 10 percent were gay men whose risk of the disease was 50 percent, as later research would show. That meant 14,500 potentially fatally ill patients for our one hundred medical beds, and we began to see a flood of cases. The patients presented not just with the Kaposi's sarcoma or pneumocystis pneumonia we already knew were typical of AIDS, but also with other strange, previously rare diseases I had never seen or expected to see.

They would come in infected by every imaginable organism—viruses, bacteria, fungi, and parasites that were supposed to stay where they belonged, in the gastrointestinal tract or on the skin, but in these patients were everywhere, in their lungs, livers, eyes, and brains. They had cancers of incredible rapidity and virulence. There was a weird, rapidly progressive dementia, which differed completely from what we were used to seeing in the elderly. Sometimes the patients would come in with fevers, and we couldn't find what was causing the fevers at all, or with a strange wasting where they would get thinner and thinner, as if they were being consumed from within.

And although we now knew the cause, we still didn't yet have a diagnostic test or any specific treatment. It was very nineteenth-century in that regard. So we did what we had been trained to do. We transfused our patients for their anemia, gave them dialysis for their renal failure, surgerized and chemotherapied their cancers, and treated their infections with antibiotics, all the time knowing it was hopeless. We did CPR and ran a Code Blue on everyone, although we assumed the disease was contagious.

How contagious?

No one knew. We didn't know, no one did, whether it might turn into Camus's Plague, worldwide and fatal. Since the government was terrified of doctors leaving the ship before it sank, it declared that the new disease was "not very contagious." We didn't have to worry about touching our patients, although we might want to wear gloves; or about respiratory secretions, although we might want to put on a mask; or about door-knobs or tables, although the virus survived on surfaces for a week.

To us interns and residents it didn't matter anyway. We were sur-rounded by blood, phlegm, and bodily excretions, we were exhausted and vulnerable, and we did what we knew how to do. We drew blood, stuck needles into arms and legs, veins and arteries, lungs, abdomens, spines; and we examined, listened, and touched. We saw so many sick young men, coughing, vomiting, scared. I began to have more sympathy for history, for those long-ago doctors presented with a new disease—malaria, plague, syphilis, the green sickness, shell shock—who, not knowing what it was, understood and treated it with the concepts and treatments they had.

In any case, there wasn't much we could do. They were so terribly sick, so terribly young and handsome. And there were so many of them, every day, with their rashes, coughs, and red eyes, their confu-sion, their fevers. We treated them the way we treated anyone, except that our most important logical principle for diagnosis, Ockham's razor, didn't work.

William of Ockham was a fourteenth-century philosopher who, in order to prove God's existence, proposed that of two possible explana-tions the simpler should be preferred. In medicine this means that we look for a single unifying diagnosis. But with AIDS, that didn't work. A patient with a fever, cough, rash, and diarrhea did not necessarily have a single diagnosis but could have three separate diagnoses all at once—pneumocystis pneumonia, cryptococcal diarrhea, and Kaposi's sarcoma, too.

You could say it was the perfect storm—an untreatable, contagious fatal disease meets Fast Medicine in the context of Free Love. And the handsomer the patient, the sooner he was infected, being the most popular in the bathhouses, and the sooner he died. I'd never imagined a dying worse than cancer, and now here it was.

But the handsomest and saddest of all was Nurse David.

Nurse David looked like Dr. Kildare in his prime, like Peter O'Toole as Lawrence of Arabia, like Leslie Howard in *Gone with the Wind*. Like a movie star.

He was medium height, trim, and carried himself high. Blond hair cut short, and clean-shaven, he was "Nurse David" in the emergency room when being a male nurse was unusual. His friends and lovers and ex-lovers came through that emergency room, sick unto death, with this new disease, by then identified as viral and infectious. Still, Nurse David did not use gloves or mask. When they came in covered with blood from vomiting or diarrhea, he cleaned them up, bare; he suctioned the mucus from their tracheas with uncovered face, he cradled their Kaposi's sarcoma heads in his arms. He was fearless and kind.

But then, when the diagnostic antibody test arrived, Nurse David disappeared from the ER, and I heard through the grapevine that he had tested positive for the AIDS virus. There was still no treatment for it, so it was a death sentence and a dying sentence, also a no-loving, no-fun sentence, if you had integrity. We all knew that condoms broke and Safe Sex was only Safer Sex: not safe enough.

I missed him.

The months passed.

And then there he was, back in the hospital but now as a patient. It was a gray late afternoon, Thanksgiving Day; I was the resident in charge of the ICU, and Nurse David's diagnosis was pneumocystis pneumonia that had failed every treatment.

Now, *Pneumocystis carinii* is a slimy, single-celled parasite that normally does live in our lungs, but just a few of them. With AIDS and the viral destruction of our T cells, though, the few parasites normally in the lungs can get out of control, like gophers in an untended lawn. They start to grow, unmolested by the body's immune system, and then divide and multiply until they fill up the honeycombs of alveoli in the lungs, and oxygen can no longer get into the bloodstream, and the patient dies of suffocation. Although we do have antibiotics that kill the parasites, for Nurse David they had already failed and we had nothing else, as he knew very well.

After he had settled into his room, I went in to see him. It was a big room with three other beds, all empty, and there were his friends all around, standing at his head, his sides, and his feet. To get oxygen into his lungs past the *Pneumocystis*, he'd been put on a respirator with a tube down his throat, so he couldn't speak, and he was being breathed by the machine with difficulty. He was covered with sweat, and even with the respirator at 100 percent oxygen, the oxygen level in his blood was below the minimum for sustained life, which is 60.

He was dying and his friends were keeping watch.

He was conscious but not very conscious, and as handsome and golden-haired as ever. He was struggling, he was waiting, there was nothing left for us to do. He was well cared for by the calmness of his friends; it was as old-fashioned a dying as there could be. Unusually for the time, he had Advanced Life Directives, and they were clear. No blood drawing. No Code Blue. No CPR. No fuss.

The ICU nurses, who were also his friends, came in now and then to check up on him. I did, too, throughout the afternoon and evening.

His breathing got worse and worse, and by eleven p.m. he was no longer conscious. He was still sweating and a little restless, stirring now and then; his oxygen level had dropped below 50, and his EKG monitor was beginning to show the ventricular heartbeats that signal the end. His friends remained calm.

The ventricular beats became more and more frequent, and then suddenly they took over David's heart rhythm as ventricular tachycardia, which cannot maintain the blood pressure, and the blood pressure began to fall. By this time, his eyes had closed and he was still, and all of us began focusing on the monitor. We watched in silence as the regular jagged beats of ventricular tachycardia degenerated into the chaotic, pre-death line of coarse ventricular fibrillation, which then became softer, smoother, and curvier until it was just a sinuous green wave flowing across the screen.

Then the wave began to flatten as it flowed, until finally it was just a single green line moving across the screen. We'd already turned off the alarms, and I checked his pulse. No pulse. I open his eyelids and checked his pupils. They were fixed and dilated.

We turned off the respirator. It was right before midnight.

But the heart monitor was still on, and I saw to my surprise over the next ten minutes, as we stood around his body which we were not yet ready to leave, an occasional normal heartbeat pop up into that flat green line. What did that mean? David was dead, and yet somewhere there was life within him still. Is that how it always goes? I wondered, but we never get to see it—sparks of life flashing out after what we call death? And in the brain and mind, too?

I thought about Henry VIII and all those severed heads being lifted up after execution; they must still have had blips going across their screens, too. And how in the nineteenth century a cord was attached to the inside of coffins and a bell outside, so that, should a corpse awaken, he would be able to signal that he was alive, the nineteenth-century rationalists being surprisingly worried about continued consciousness in a dead body.

It took ten minutes for those thought-blips to stop interrupting that flowing flat green line.

Then I turned off the monitor and went to see my next patient.

That was what the AIDS epidemic was like, if you were a second-year medical resident in the eye of the eye of the storm.

I was exhausted, depressed, and in despair, and I decided to quit. I couldn't see how I could manage for another year and a half. I didn't want to quit but I couldn't imagine how I could maintain my Self. And then came Turnaround Month, and I didn't quit, and it was all because of what happened in the emergency room.

You wouldn't have thought so—the ER, rough, quick, brutal; in the waiting room, standing-room only and sometimes the line went out the door into the street. Its cubicles and gurneys were always filled, and so was the blackboard with the names in chalk of the patients waiting to be seen by the internal medicine resident. Each patient took two hours to examine and triage, and on a bad day, there could be six patients on that blackboard, which meant twelve hours, with more patients being added as those hours went by. It was impossible and hopeless, if you did the math. On my worst day I admitted nineteen patients and filled up the entire ICU.

It was endless, though not always thankless, and certainly unsatisfying; it was the pool with the hole you're always trying to fill up in Algebra 3. There were cuts, scrapes, accidents; heart failure and heart attacks; dementia and delirium and dehydration; chest pain, head pain, foot pain, and abdominal pain; seizures, cancers, pneumonias, and psychoses.

I was oppressed, suppressed, repressed, and depressed and I couldn't stand my fresh-faced, eager, good-looking interns any longer. I couldn't stand the ER docs, especially Dr. Dobbins, who was shabby and overweight with a round face, sketchy beard, and acne scars, and who turfed his inadequately worked-up patients so cheerfully to us medical residents. It seemed to me that everything we did was wasted—the men with AIDS died of their AIDS a few months later than they would have without us, and those were months of torture. Ditto the cirrhotics with their bleeding, the diabetics with their gangrenous legs, the cancer patients with their chemotherapy, the demented patients with their pneumonias.

But this month was Turnaround Month.

Turnaround Month was the month of residency when, instead of working as a second-year resident, I would act as a third-year resident.

It provided a way to experience the role we would be playing the next year, but under the direction of someone who was already doing it. It meant that I would be running the Code Blues, doing the surgical consultations, and being responsible for the hospital, while the third-year resident would be acting as the second-year resident—admitting the patients, teaching the interns, and doing most of the work. So it was bad news, good news. But the best news of all was that the third-year resident for the month was Dr. Annie Leeds. This was the best news because Dr. Annie Leeds was perfect, and I'm not even being ironic.

She was beautiful, for starters. She had a shapely body, prematurely gray hair with the blue-gray eyes that go along with that, and unlined skin. What's more, she was always, improbably, impeccably dressed, in skirt, nylons, heels, an unwrinkled blouse and stylish jacket, with makeup perfectly applied, even at three a.m. No one knew how she did it. Plus, she was cheerful, knowledgeable, and mature.

It was our first night on call together and we had our two interns with us, one of whom I particularly didn't like. Big and strong, Mike had curly reddish hair, a square jaw, flat face, and freckles, and he was Midwest-polite, deferential but cold. He had a kind of eye-rolling about him, a waiting, a hidden impatience for the year to be over and he could take his rightful place as man in charge, as second-year resident. So I thought.

It was eight-thirty p.m., and Annie suggested we all go down to the conference room for pizza. She'd already ordered it. We sat at the long table and the pizza arrived. But next to us, on the other side of the open partition, there was an AA meeting going on and it was noisy and I got up to close the pleated steel partition between us. I pulled it and it stretched, unfurled, snapped open, and then accordioned onto my left hand, which disappeared into a steel pleat. I pulled it open and got out my hand, now covered with blood and with my fingers missing. I stared at the hand for a second. It was a bloody stump. It was my left hand, and I thought—and this will give you some idea of how tired we all were, how off—Oh well. Looks like I amputated my fingers. Guess I'll need to get a dressing before seeing my next patient.

I turned around to tell Annie, and found her, Mike, and the other intern, Jason, staring at my hand, aghast.

"You need to go to the ER," said Annie.

"Why bother?" I told her. "I've had a tetanus shot." That's how whacked I was. And already it was starting to be clear that the fingers hadn't been amputated, just crushed, and now they were reappearing as a bloody pulpy mess.

Annie got up. So did Mike and Jason. "We're going with you to the ER. Put your hand up," Annie instructed.

I held my hand up and it dripped blood as we walked over to the elevator. Mike pushed the button. We waited until the doors opened and then stepped in.

I opened my eyes. Dr. Dobbins was leaning over me. His face was concerned and kind.

"What happened?" I asked him.

"You passed out in the elevator," he said. "They thought you'd coded. Mike picked you up and carried you here. We've already done the X-ray—no fractures. We've cleaned your hand, and now I'm getting ready to sew it up."

There was an IV going into my left arm—how did they do that without me knowing?—and I was wearing a hospital gown and lying on a gurney looking up into the fluorescent light of the ER's room 5. Then Dr. Dobbins gave me the gentlest of injections and began sewing up my fingers. Expertly, with full attention. The wounded surgeon plied the steel, which questioned—actually repaired—the distempered—actually crushed—part. Beneath his bleeding hands—actually my bleeding hand—I felt the sharp compassion of the healer's art. So saith T. S. Eliot.

After Dr. Dobbins was done, he pushed away the tray and began dressing my hand with sterile four-by-fours. Then he wrapped it up. It didn't hurt.

"Annie says you should go home. Do you need someone to drive you?"

"Who's going to do my work?"

"She will."

"I feel fine," I said. "It's just my left hand."

"Do you want some Tylenol with codeine?"

"No. Maybe some Tylenol."

"I'll let the bag of IV fluid run in, then. And I'll tell Annie."

Dr. Dobbins left.

I lay there alone, staring at the ceiling, looking at the IV drip, and wondering how they got my shirt off; how all these things had happened with my not knowing, not being active or helpful, but passive, unconscious, a patient. Then the nurse came in.

It was Marge, who was an old-fashioned nurse, hard-bitten, tough. She told me once that no one should die alone, and if a patient was dying, or already dead, she would stay with him for a while even after her shift was done.

"How did you get my shirt off?" I asked, as she was cleaning up.

"Oh, we had to cut it off."

"I can't remember anything."

"You were out."

The IV was finished and she took it out and put a Band-Aid on my left antecubital fossa. "You should stay a while longer."

"My beeper keeps going off. I feel okay."

I got up slowly and watched my world go from horizontal to vertical, from being a patient to being a doctor; from passive to active; from being taken care of to taking care of.

I answered my page.

"Where have you been?!" said Terry, the ICU intern. "I've been paging you for an hour! I'm all alone up here in the ICU."

"I'll be up."

My left hand was wrapped but I wasn't unsteady and it hadn't yet begun to hurt. I started out of the ER, and as I got to the door, Mike appeared.

"You're okay!" he said. "You passed out in the elevator! We stepped in with you; there were other people in it; it started, and you turned pale—white!—and went down. I thought we'd have to call a code. We couldn't get a pulse; but then the door opened to the ER and I picked you up and carried you in. . . . You were so light! You didn't weigh anything at all!"

He looked at me, and I looked at him, and we both measured how we would manage this new relationship. We would put it away, we decided silently, somewhere else.

"Thank you," I said, and went upstairs to the ICU to see how bad things were.

They were pretty bad, but that was the turning point for me, that turn-around from doctor to patient.

In Hebrew there is a concept called *teshuvah*, usually translated as "repentance" but which actually means "turning" or "returning." It is the task for the ten-day interval between the Jewish New Year, when the Book of Fate is opened, and Yom Kippur, when it is closed, and it implies a re-thinking, a re-solving, a re-turning to what is important in life. So it's turning a new leaf or turning a page or turning on your heel. It's changing direction—being certain of the view in front of you, then turning around and seeing a different view, which was always there but now you've turned around and seen it.

What I had seen before, in front of me, were the failings of Dr. Dobbins and Mike and the hospital itself. But now on Turnaround Day I saw that their failings were personal and contingent but their success was archetypal.

"Archetype" is the name Jung gave to those complexes of thoughts, feelings, and images that arise cross-culturally, independent of direct transmission. That was, he thought, because they come out of the fundamental nature of being human. There is, for example, the archetype of Mother, the archetype of Child, the archetype of Wholeness. Jung believed that much of our inner world is structured by these unconscious archetypes—the desires they arise from, the expectations they create, and the needs they satisfy.

And for me on Turnaround Day, what I understood was the archetypal nature of Medicine. Dr. Dobbins leaning over, sewing up my wound, was not only Dr. Dobbins; he was also, mainly, the Doctor—kind, objective, competent. Annie Leeds was Older Sister, Mike was the Prince who saved me from the Dragon, and the hospital was not simply a Factory for Healing; it was also, mainly, a Place for the Care of Those Who Can't Take Care of Themselves.

The hospital, too, had failings. It could be taken over, its purpose subverted and turned upside down, but even then, that didn't change the amazing fact of its success, its being. Behind the hospital of steel and glass I knew so well was another hospital, an archetypical place that answered the question: Where do I go when I'm sick and helpless? A mystical hospital that does not need steel and glass, although steel and glass need it; that would exist even if it moved out of doors and set up shop in the parking lot.

That mystical hospital, I realized on Turnaround Day, as I felt myself a patient, unable to take care of myself, is made up of doctors and nurses, and their caring, skills, and competence. Without them and those, all the shiny technology, the IV and sterile saline, the beautiful steel needles in their aluminum packets, the Xylocaine and Betadine, would have sat on the steel tray next to my gurney, useless and unused.

So when I stood up, when I turned from horizontal to vertical, from patient to doctor, I found that my perspective had changed. I was a wounded healer, and there was much more to the hospital than appeared. From then on, although I would still be exhausted, depressed, and frustrated, I would be aware, even at the worst of times—four a.m., with no sleep and a screaming patient, a dying patient, an anxious nurse, and a tricky procedure to do—that I could key into the mystical hospital that lay behind the material hospital.

Not *key* in as in opening a locked door, but *key* in as in tuning to the right key, the key of wakefulness, the key of awakedness. Where I wasn't exhausted but clearheaded, and where my fellows were not coworkers in a factory but companions on Crusade, stopping to take care of those who had fallen in battle.

Thus I entered the archetype of Physician through the archetype of Patient.

Up to that point, though Beryl had thanked me and I had the Mantle of Hippocrates placed upon my shoulders, and had even seen Mr. Sturm come back to life, I hadn't grasped the archetype of Physician. Not until I myself became a patient, and understood from inside the archetype of Patient, which is an archetype of dependence, of helplessness and need, could I understood its opposite. It is the vulnerability, fear, and dependence of the patient that calls forth the archetype of Physician— calm, unafraid, authoritative. A call and an answer. As long as there is sickness, therefore, there will be patients, and as long as there are patients, there will be physicians.

And so I didn't quit but made it through that year and into the last year of my training, which would be a year of crystallization, when all that amorphous knowledge and experience, those hundreds of patients and thousands of experiences, would coalesce into a structure.

TWELVE

A Craft, a Science, and an Art

The third year of residency is the end of the apprenticeship, the year to become a master at Fast Medicine. By that time you are almost an expert, and you're given the most responsibility: you oversee the hospital, run the Code Blues, and take care of the ICU, and even the attendings defer to you. Your primary obligation is to pass the Medical Boards, and in the meantime you mainly act as a consultant for the different medical specialties of cardiology, nephrology, infectious disease, and so on. So it is a year of consolidating your knowledge, of almost-there. I imagine the final journeyman year of the medieval cobbler or stone mason must have been the same, with that sense of incipient freedom to practice your craft.

By then I understood that medicine is, above all, a craft.

"Craft" from the German *Kraft*—the "power that comes from knowing." The *OED* defines "craft" as "a collection of practical skills directed toward one end," but what I mean by "craft" is that you can learn it only by doing, by being taught and mentored. So it is the opposite of what you can learn on a computer, because it is about getting a feel for things. It takes a guild, therefore, to transmit a craft, a group of knowers who pass along their knowledge in a step-by-step way from simple to complex, and take pleasure in watching their students become masters themselves.

The craft of medicine is a beautiful thing, very human, very much about body, not only the patient's real bleeding body, but through and in your own body. It is what I learned by taking care of Mrs. Carmona. You can't fake it. It takes a warm human energy, a commitment, a struggle, a giving up of a piece of yourself to attain that craft.

So it was my final journeyman year, which traditionally ends with a "chef d'oeuvre," a masterwork, presented to the elder masters. The cobbler presents an elegant handmade shoe, the chef a magnificent marzipan castle, the physician a Grand Rounds—a lecture about an important patient he's taken care of, whose disease he believes the masters should learn about.

The masters circle his creation, criticize it, and, at last, nod their heads.

Thus you are accepted, you are done. You are a master, though a young master, and you can go off and deepen your craft independently. And that is what that last year of residency is really about.

But medicine is not only a craft, Mrs. Mary Mather would convince me that year. It is also the science it so wants to be—logical, at least sometimes, and for which every detail, even the most obscure, can come in handy.

I met Mrs. Mather during the month I was the senior resident for medicine, responsible for knowing all the sick patients in the hospital. It was late morning and I went over to the Step-Down Unit, a kind of lesser ICU, to hear about the newest admission from the night before.

The second-year resident told me about her. Mrs. Mather was married, fifty-five, no kids, he began, and she'd been a psychiatric nurse with a long history herself of schizophrenia and depression. Last week she'd gone to the ER for back pain, been prescribed codeine, and abruptly stopped her usual cocktails and wine when they told her not to take it with alcohol. The codeine didn't help, she went back to the ER and got Percocet, and two days later she started having grand mal seizures. Her husband brought her back to the ER, they treated the seizures, but then late last night the seizures started up again, and nothing would stop them until the anesthesiologist came in and put her under. Then this morning, her labs came back and her ammonia level was 320. So she was in liver failure. She wasn't a candidate for a liver transplant, they couldn't find her husband, and no one knew what to do. Obviously they were trying to get her ammonia level down with the usual meds, and her attending, Dr. Rose, was here now to review her case and help with decision making.

I listened. It sounded classic: Alcoholic abruptly stops drinking and starts having grand mal seizures from alcohol withdrawal, then turns out to have cirrhosis of the liver. You don't need much of your liver to survive, only about 5 percent, but without that 5 percent, you die. It's up to your liver to detoxify your blood, to produce albumin so the serum in your blood stays in your veins, and to make coagulation proteins so you don't bleed to death. I'd seen many deaths from cirrhosis by then, gruesome and unstoppable even by Fast Medicine. Suddenly the cirrhotic would sit up in bed, vomit his entire blood volume onto the sheets, and die. Or the serum in his blood would seep into his abdomen, filling it up, and then his blood pressure would slowly drop to not-enough. Or he would turn yellow and go into a hepatic coma from the ammonia his liver could no longer remove from his blood. Mrs. Mather was even more classic, because most likely she didn't have schizophrenia and depression but rather manic-depression, and had been treating both her mania and her depression over the years with alcohol.

I should go see her. She would probably die in the next few days, and I should be ready to perform her unnecessary and ineffectual Code Blue.

Then I looked down the hallway and saw Dr. Rose. He, too, was classic, though rarer. He was English, small and neat with a head of gray curls, manicured hands, and Italian shoes. He spoke with a rapid, strong English accent and his love was unusual diseases. He read the medical journals voraciously and had a tenacious memory; presiding over Morning Report, the daily gathering of hospital doctors to hear about the night's admissions, he always had some fascinating, obscure take on the cases.

Although that was certainly not why he was here today. One of his other duties as Chief of Medicine was to help us residents with difficult ethical issues; in this instance, what to do with Mrs. MM, who was going to die of liver failure.

I walked over to him, said hi, and then looked inside Mrs. MM's room. She was alone, a mound of bedclothes being breathed by a respirator. I went in to get a better look. I stood by her bed and looked down.

Mrs. MM was lying quite still, deeply asleep. Her eyes were closed, her face slack, and she had the pursed-out lips of the respirator-breathed comatose patient. Her nose was fleshy, her face swollen, her brown hair short and badly cut. Her arms were outside the bedcovers; I lifted her right arm up to feel its tone, and it fell back to the bed with a thud.

I thought about liver failure. Mrs. Mather's liver should have been filtering out the ammonia our body makes out of the protein we eat, and then sending it to the kidney to be excreted in the urine. But instead, her ammonia level had gotten so high that it had caused intractable seizures and now coma. Without a liver transplant, she would never wake up.

I stood there and looked at her for a while.

And suddenly I noticed something strange about her. She wasn't yellow, and she should have been yellow, very yellow. When the liver fails and stops being able to detoxify ammonia, it also stops being able to detoxify the bilirubin from the hemoglobin of used-up blood. So as the ammonia level rises, so does the bilirubin level, and it turns the skin yellow. I opened Mrs. Mather's eyes to be sure. The whites of her eyes were white.

This was very strange.

Then I threw off her covers to examine her thoroughly. Patients with liver failure also get "spider angiomata"—little red spots of broken blood vessels—but Mrs. Mather didn't have any. She didn't have any bruises either, which occur when the liver stops producing coagulation proteins.

Then I checked her liver and spleen. In liver failure the liver can either be enlarged or very small, but hers was normal in size and texture. I couldn't feel her spleen either, and it should, in liver failure, be palpable. Nor was her abdomen swollen with fluid, nor her legs edematous.

Weird. I could find no signs of liver failure on Mrs. Mather's body, and yet her ammonia level was the highest I'd ever seen.

It didn't make sense. And although over the years I'd not been impressed with the perfect logic of the body, if the scientific method worked at all in medicine, Mrs. Mather's ammonia level would have to make sense.

So I went through the steps of the scientific method.

First. Confirm the finding.

I left Mrs. MM's room, got her chart, and went over her labs. Except for her ammonia level, they were all normal. Liver enzymes, clotting factors, albumin—all fine. There was no evidence from her labs that her liver had failed.

Second. Come up with an alternative hypothesis.

I went looking for Dr. Rose. He was in the nurses' station going over another chart, and I asked him, What did he think? If Mrs. Mather's elevated ammonia level was due to liver failure, how come all her liver functions were normal?

He looked up from his chart, put his glasses on his forehead, and replied, "Obviously she's in liver failure. The reason her liver enzymes are normal is because her liver is so dead it has no enzymes left—you know that."

"Yeah, but everything except the ammonia is normal. Not only her enzymes, but her bilirubin, albumin, and clotting factors are normal. Except for the ammonia level, there isn't any evidence she has liver failure."

Dr. Rose thought for a bit. Then,

"Porto-systemic shunt," he nodded to himself. "That must be it. She must be bypassing her liver. There was just such a case two years ago where there was an intrahepatic shunt. Fascinating. The ammoniated blood can't get to the liver and so it builds up in the blood and causes hepatic coma."

Now, I'd always respected Dr. Rose's rare cases, but I couldn't see how this one would fit Mrs. MM's bill. An "intrahepatic shunt" means an unusual connection between one of the arteries in the liver, bringing toxic blood in, and a vein, bringing usually cleansed blood out. A "shunt" means a bypass. Dr. Rose was suggesting that Mrs. MM had suddenly developed such a connection, and that a large portion of her toxified ammoniated blood was bypassing the liver instead of getting detoxified by the liver. Hence the elevated ammonia level.

But if that were the case, I asked, shouldn't Mrs. MM also be yellow? Bilirubin was another toxic product, and it should also be bypassing the liver.

He listened, shook his head, put his glasses back on, and went back to reading his chart.

For the rest of that day, Mrs. MM's ammonia continued to rise, astronomically. Normal ammonia level is less than 40, and her first level of 320 was the highest I'd ever seen. But Mrs. MM's ammonia did not stop there. The next one was 480 and then 562, and no one had ever seen a level that high. But she still wasn't yellow, not even a bit; her liver enzymes stayed normal and her albumin didn't fall, nor did her coagulation proteins. Something else was up.

So, third: When all else fails, go to the library.

Since I wasn't a second-year resident trapped by an overwhelming number of patients but a third-year resident, a gentleman doctor despite my gender, in the late afternoon I left the hospital and went over to the university library. If ever medicine should prove itself a science, Mrs. Mather's sky-high ammonia level had to make sense.

How could an ammonia level rise to toxic levels in the face of a normal liver?

Suddenly I remembered something from those first few months of medical school. Biochemistry. We'd had to memorize the cell cycles—the cytochrome cycle, the ATP cycle—the consecutive enzymes of how the body makes energy out of glucose, how it disposes of carbon dioxide. At the time, it seemed arcane, unnecessary, and indeed in the future all that memorization would be cut out of the medical curriculum. But I was glad I'd learned it, because there it was when I needed it—the urea cycle.

The urea cycle is a series of enzymes in the liver that consecutively removes ammonia from the blood, attaches it to a molecule of carbon dioxide to form urea, and then sends the urea to the kidney to be excreted in the urine. And I wondered: Could Mrs. MM have a failure not of her liver but of her urea cycle?

Did that ever happen?

I began to take down books from the bookshelves as the afternoon faded.

It did happen by three different mechanisms, I learned: a toxin, a poison, or a genetic defect.

Fourth, narrow down the possibilities.

The urea cycle could be stopped by certain toxins. For instance, in China in the 1950s there'd been a brief epidemic of urea-cycle poisoning due to a batch of spoiled soy. Also there were certain fish that produce a toxin which can block the urea cycle. There was even a drying agent added to cake mixes in the 1930s that blocked the urea cycle. I wondered: Could Mrs. MM have found an aging—very aged—box of brownie mix? At a garage sale, perhaps? Her ill-cut hair had me imagining her coming home with a cheap box of brownie mix, making it, and . . . seizing. Okay, far-fetched. Toxins seemed unlikely and I crossed them off my list.

Could Mrs. MM have been poisoned? Her husband worked in a lab, I'd heard, and I read about a chemical called "jackbean urease," which was frequently used in labs to block the urea cycle. I was sure Mrs. MM hadn't been easy to live with all those years, what with her drinking and depressions. Poison seemed unlikely but not impossible, so I kept it on my list but moved it lower.

Last, what about a genetic defect in her urea cycle?

There was one possibility. It was in the urea cycle enzyme known as ornithine transcarbamylase, or OTC. Its gene was on the X chromosome, and so males, with their XY configuration, have only one copy of it, but females, who are XX, have two copies. Consequently, male infants born with a defective OTC gene cannot process ammonia at all and die early, usually as infants, from intractable seizures. But females do pretty well, because, with their extra copy of the OTC gene, they produce enough OTC to detoxify their ammonia, until they get sick. Then their ammonia levels do get very high and cause episodes of confusion, psychosis, or seizures.

If that was what Mrs. MM had, it would explain not only her present condition but her whole sad life. If she was heterozygous for OTC deficiency, then all her life she would have been having episodes of sky-high ammonia, where she would get confused and hallucinate, and which would have gotten her that diagnosis of schizophrenia. The current episode would have been set off by the narcotics for her back pain, which would have interfered with the half dose of OTC she usually made and tipped her into hyperammonemia and intractable seizures.

If so, what would happen now if we could get the ammonia out of her body—with dialysis, say? Would she wake up? Would she be fine?

I decided to ask Dr. Rose.

So the next morning I went looking for him and found him outside her room, writing a note.

I asked him, Could Mrs. Mather be heterozygous for an OTC deficiency? Wouldn't that explain her high ammonia level and normal liver? If so, couldn't we treat it with dialysis?

It wouldn't matter, he said. Her ammonia level this morning was 818 and she was brain-dead. He shook his head. All those seizures. He just wished they could find her husband.

But ammonia doesn't actually injure the brain, I said. Maybe if we got the ammonia out with dialysis, she'd wake up.

He shook his head again. "It's the seizures. And now she fulfills all the Harvard criteria for brain death. Both of her EEGs are flat, she has no cold calorics, and she failed the apnea test. She's brain-dead and I'm ordering the respirator turned off this afternoon."

"But couldn't the ammonia and the anesthesia interfere with those tests? How do we know her EEG is really flat?"

"She's in liver failure," he said, and finished writing his order.

"Well, then, can I get tests for OTC deficiency anyway?"

"Yes. Yes, you may. Go ahead."

Mrs. Mather's husband never did show up, and her respirator was turned off that afternoon. But before that, I did send off those labs. If ever medicine was a science, I knew, they had to show heterozygous OTC deficiency.

I knew also that if I'd been in Dr. Rose's place, I wouldn't have ordered the respirator turned off without a trial of dialysis. Probably I would have been wrong. Probably her brain was indeed mush after all those seizures, and most likely it would have been another disaster, as with Mrs. Carmona, of technology keeping a body alive when it shouldn't be. But still. I would have tried, in spite of her no cold calorics and flat EEG and Harvard criteria, just in case medicine was also, at the same time—not a science.

Mrs. Mather's blood and tissue would go to a genetics lab and take two months to come back, and in the meantime, I would meet my patient Mr. Danska. Ours would be a short-term relationship, just a one-night stand, but it would get me thinking about how medicine was not only a craft and a science but also an art. That it had something unexplainable about it, which was its heart.

The case of Mr. Danska started one night when I was on call for the ICU, resting in the tiny airless call room reserved for the senior medical resident. Bare walls, a single bed in the corner, next to which was a chair with a phone on it. No windows. If it had been a prison cell, the State would have sued. And we were always so happy to be inside it.

I was lying on the bed, eyes closed. It was only nine p.m., but I'd learned to take my rest when I could get it. My beeper went off. It was the ER and I called back.

"Hey, this is Dr. S. Did someone beep me?"

"Yeah, I did. It's Dobbins. I've got an admission for you. Guy, forty-two years old, having an anterior MI. Pain pretty well controlled with morphine and nitrates, but he's having runs of v-tach. I've got him on max lidocaine and amiodarone, but they're still coming, and we had to shock him once already here. You need to come down and escort him up to the ICU."

"Okay, be right down."

I left the call room, went downstairs, and found Mr. Danska lying on a gurney in the hallway with his head elevated. He was a small, slim man, not the type of frame you'd expect to be having a massive heart attack, and with thinning blond hair. He had oxygen going, an IV in each arm, and an EKG monitor next to him. He was pale under his tan, drawn but calm.

"Hi. I'm Dr. S and this is the intern, Ron. We'll be taking you up to the ICU. How're you doing?"

Mr. D smiled. "All right," he said, in an accent I couldn't place.

"How's the pain?"

"Not bad."

"Where are you from?"

"Burlingame," he said with a tired twinkle.

"No, originally."

"Denmark."

We rolled Mr. D out of the ER toward the elevator, and I continued to distract him with chitchat. The elevator doors opened. It was empty, and we three got in. The intern pushed 7 and the doors closed.

It was quiet. The elevator started to go up. Suddenly . . .

"Damn."

"What?" the intern asked.

"Look at the monitor," I said. "He's in v-tach." "V-tach" is ventricular tachycardia, a rapid heart rate that arises from a damaged left ventricle and can turn quickly into ventricular fibrillation, a pre-death rhythm.

"Should we shock him?"

I was watching the monitor and Mr. D. "Not yet."

Then Mr. D's eyes closed and his head dropped back. The elevator stopped at 4 and the doors opened but no one got in. The doors closed.

Mr. D was now unconscious. But I didn't want to shock him. We were alone in an elevator—anything could happen. He could flatline, and then what were we going to do? So I decided to try carotid sinus massage.

The way carotid sinus massage works is that the carotid sinus is in the carotid artery, which takes blood from the heart to the brain. It is a small group of pressure-sensitive cells in a little pouch, or sinus, and it regulates the pulse, fast or slow depending on the blood pressure it senses in the artery. If the blood pressure is low, it speeds up the heart; if the blood pressure is high, it slows down the pulse. The idea behind carotid massage is that rubbing the carotid artery at the level of the carotid sinus puts pressure on those cells; they sense the blood pressure as being high, and therefore, they slow the pulse down. It is a mechanical, not a chemical or electrical way, to slow or sometimes even convert a rapid cardiac rhythm.

I'd learned it as a medical student. There had been two of us and our resident showed us how to do it and then told us to go over to a patient in the ICU and try it. We each stood on one side of the patient, put our respective fingers on the carotid sinus of the left and the right, and rubbed, and the patient's heart slowed down so much that it stopped. The alarms all went off, our resident came running and told us never, ever, to rub both carotid sinuses at once. We took our fingers off and the patient's heart started up again.

So I knew it did work.

I put two fingers on the right side of Mr. D's neck where the carotid sinus should be and then rubbed pretty hard. And sure enough, as I was rubbing and watching, the monitor showed the green sawtooth line of v-tach slowing, then stopping and going flat for a second, and then starting up again in a perfect normal sinus rhythm. A few seconds later, Mr. D woke up, and the elevator doors opened. We wheeled him through the double doors of the ICU into his room and then turned him over to the care of the ICU nurses. That was always a relief, because the ICU nurses were amazing. They were with their cardiac patients all day and all night, and had tricks we doctors didn't even dream of.

I went back to the call room, which was right next to the ICU, and lay down on the bed. Sometime later, the phone rang. It was Linda, Mr. D's nurse.

"Hi, Dr. S, sorry to wake you up, but Mr. D is back in v-tach. Would you come over and take a look? He's dropped his pressure twenty points and is out of it."

"Sure."

I got up, went into the ICU, and found Mr. D. He was out of it all right. Unconscious and his blood pressure was down to 80. I checked the monitor. Yes, it was v-tach.

"Shall I get the paddles?" asked Linda.

"Wait a minute. I tried carotid massage in the elevator and it worked. I'm gonna try it again."

I stood on Mr. D's right, draped my fingers around his neck, and rubbed, again, for ten seconds. The sawtooth green line of v-tach slowed, stretched out, stopped, flatlined, and then resumed as a normal sinus rhythm.

"How are his lytes?" I asked.

"All fine. He's on morphine, nitrates, antiarrhythmics, of course, oxygen, and good pain control. BP is okay, now."

"Okay. Good. Nothing much else to do. But why don't I show you what I did in case he goes into v-tach again?"

"Great. No one has ever shown me before."

I demonstrated—not on Mr. D. I didn't want his pulse to slow any more. I pointed. "Press here. It's a kind of firm rubbing, like this. Got it?"

"I think so. Hope you get a good rest-of-the-night sleep."

"Thanks."

I did fall asleep but soon there was a knock on the door and a quiet voice.

"Dr. S, sorry to bother you again, but he's back in v-tach and I tried carotid massage but it didn't work."

"Okay, no problem, I'll be over."

By now it was two a.m., and Mr. D was looking pretty tired and wan. He, too, was worried. But he was awake.

"Hi, Mr. D. How're you doing? How's the pain?"

"It's okay. It's better. But I can feel that fluttering in my chest. Are you going to shock me?"

"Well, maybe. Let's see." I stood there and draped my fingers over his neck and rubbed his carotid, and he converted again, from v-tach to normal sinus. He could feel the difference from the inside and smiled up at me.

"Thanks."

"Don't mention it."

Then Linda asked, "How come I couldn't do that? Show me again, will you? And let me get one of the other nurses so she can see." She went out.

Mr. D and I stayed together for a while. We were both tired and quiet, but somehow companionable. Mr. D trusted me by this time, he trusted my fingers, and he relaxed. I looked at his relaxed though tired face and thought how much I liked the Danes. They were cool in World War II, clever. Other countries fought for their Jews or surrendered them, but the Danes simply put on yellow stars regardless, including the king, and so you couldn't tell who was who.

Linda returned with Karen, and I gave them a demonstration. I drew an X over the spot on Mr. D's neck. "This is where the carotid sinus is, more or less. Stand on the right side, drape your fingers over, and rub, like this, maybe for ten seconds. This amount of pressure . . ."

I leaned across the bed and rubbed Linda's forearm.

Linda and Karen nodded. They got it. It wasn't difficult.

I left and went back to my call room and fell asleep around three a.m. But soon after, there was a whisper at the door.

"It's Linda. I'm sorry, Dr. S, but we both tried, and it didn't work."

I got up, went in, massaged Mr. D's neck, and he converted. And so it went for the rest of the night. About every half an hour Mr. D went into v-tach, and my fingers converted him back. I didn't mind. But I did wonder why such a wonderful ICU nurse as Linda couldn't do the same thing. Strange.

Around five a.m., Mr. D went to sleep. His pain had resolved; his MI had ended; and the irritable area of his heart, neither completely dead nor completely alive, that had been causing all those episodes of v-tach, relaxed, too. There were no more calls to the call room, and I, too, slept.

Two weeks later, it was the day of Mr. Danska's discharge. Since our night together, we hadn't seen each other but I'd heard he'd done well. He was walking without pain, without oxygen, and his wife came in and took him home. But that afternoon, a box was delivered to the operator's cubbyhole and she called me.

"Dr. S? It's the operator. A florist just delivered a box for you. . . . No, no card . . . I don't know . . . Well, you'll have to come down and get it before I leave at five."

Later in the day, when everything was quiet, I went to get it. I walked down the stairs, thinking about Mr. D, his heart, and my fingers. I was remembering that no matter how well I tried to teach those amazing nurses to massage his carotid sinus, his heart responded only to my touch.

What was that about, really?

I recalled one of my favorite attendings, Dr. Towie Fong, and how I once saw him stop a patient's continuous seizures with his hands—by touching. He laughed a little self-consciously when he saw me notice, then lifted up his hands, showed them to me, and said, "These hands, Victoria! These hands!"

I wasn't sure what he meant by that. I did not think Mr. D's heart had something to do with my hands. It was simply that my fingers knew where to go and how to press; they just knew. It wasn't a healing touch. It was more the way a good cook knows to put a little more salt in the broth without even tasting, or a really good gardener stops at a plant, adjusts its leaves, and gives it a smidgeon of water. My fingers just knew. It was something extra, almost unnamable, just a feeling.

I knocked on the operator's door, and she handed me the long white box that had been crowding her cubbyhole all afternoon.

I stood outside her door and opened it. Inside, nestled in soft white tissue, were one dozen long-stemmed red roses.

They were an answer and a message, and the absence of a card confirmed the message. Mr. Danska knew I would know who sent them, for the same reason he sent them. Which was that we had connected, and it was that personal connection his carotid sinus responded to.

They were the answer to my question, "What was that about?"

Medicine, those roses told me, was not only a craft but also an art because, like any true art, it is based on love between subject and object—between a painter and his canvas, a sculptor and his stone, a writer and his words. That didn't mean that medicine wasn't also a craft. It certainly was a craft because it was a skill—many skills, acquired over thousands of hours and thousands of patients. But it was also an art because there was that seventh sense to it—knowing where to put my fingers, or rather, my fingers knowing where to go.

Art is what you can't teach. I just knew and felt exactly where "it"— the right place to press—was, even though anatomy has never been my forte, and I can't tell you without looking it up where exactly the carotid sinus is. But I can see and feel, to this day, exactly where and how much to press on Mr. Danska's neck. I "had a feel" for it. That "feel" was made up of that personal connection, acknowledged by those red roses, without a card but with confidence they didn't need a card. Roses—the personal, the intimate, the face-to-face—and art—the extra, that separates it from craft—in a long white box, like a beating heart in a living body.

The report of Mrs. Mather's OTC test finally arrived. It was conclusive—her level of OTC was less than half the normal level, which meant she was indeed heterozygous for OTC and medicine was not only a craft and an art but also a science.

What was too bad was that it had never been diagnosed while she was alive. If she'd only known, she could have been careful about her protein intake, since it is the protein we eat that makes the ammonia, and when she got confused and began to hallucinate, instead of getting the life-limiting diagnosis of schizophrenia, her ammonia level could have been treated. We know now that the diagnosis of heterozygous OTC deficiency is not uncommon, and an ammonia level is not an expensive test.

Dr. Rose let me give my Grand Rounds, my masterwork, on Mrs. Mather and her unusual but not rare disease, alerting everyone to its possibility. The masters milled around for a while, they looked at it from all directions, prodded, murmured, and finally nodded and accepted. I was done with my training, they agreed, I finally had Fast Medicine under my belt.

I was now a master, though a young master, and my medical exploring could begin.

THIRTEEN

Upstairs, Downstairs

The very same month in which I gave my Grand Rounds, Carlo Petrini in Italy announced the founding of the "Slow Food Movement." He was the perfect person to have done so.

Petrini was an ex-Berkeleyite Italian, who, after getting flavored himself by Berkeley's counterculture, returned to his hometown, Bra, in Piedmont, and was horrified to discover its infiltration by American culture. When, shortly thereafter, McDonald's announced it was building a Golden Arches in Rome, in protest he organized a festival of cooking and eating named "Slow Food." This was in opposition to Fast Food, "fast" being the defining principle of postwar American pride; fast! with its implication of modernity, excitement, and efficiency, as opposed to "slow"—behind the times, lumbering, inefficient, everything that business did not want to be.

Petrini's "slow" picked up on the organic food movement, and those other strains that had been brewing around me so long ago, of individuality, sensuality, and rebellion. It was an *enantiodromia* that Jung would have appreciated—of opposites giving birth to one another—slow giving birth to fast giving birth to slow. Opposites contain one another, he believed, and structures, even thought-structures, move to equilibrium. Anything that is "too much" engenders an opposite counterbalance; the pendulum reaches its furthest point and swings back in the opposite direction with the exact same force.

"Slow" therefore caught on, and Petrini began to create other Slow Food events—feasts, conventions, seminars, an international organization, even a manifesto. It would be a long time before Slow would make its way to Medicine, however, in part because who, at first thought, would want slow surgery, a slow hospital, or a slow doctor? It would take years for the charm of Fast Medicine to wear off, to engender its own opposite— years of rush and pressure, of wrong diagnoses and wrong treatments. But once this engendering began, it would happen in many places, at the same time, independently. Slow Medicine would arise as a kind of antidote.

In the meantime, though, Fast Medicine had to reach its apotheosis, and would do so by creating "healthcare," for which medical care is not a craft, science, and art but a commodity, bought and sold on Wall Street.

I would first collide with its strange ideas in a remarkable clinic, which I liked as soon as I saw it.

After the residency was over, I took the summer off, studied, and passed the Internal Medicine Boards, and then looked around for a place to practice. I wanted someplace away from things, especially from Silicon Valley, which by then was exploding with ideas and ambition. I found it over the bridge and through the woods, in a rather grand clinic situated at the outskirts of the metropolis, at the border of urban, suburban, and rural. I'll call it the Big Clinic.

I got there as a locum. It needed a temporary internist and its medical director, Dr. Roark, hired me for a few months. But I ended up staying for several years. It turned out to be a lot like the little clinic with

Dr. Meryl and Ms. Jane Lloyd, but it was much bigger, with three doctors, two physician assistants, more than thirty support staff, a medical director, and an executive director. And it wasn't a County Clinic but a "Community Clinic," which, as I would find out, was a very different thing, politically.

It started in a trailer as a free clinic. But by the time I got there, it was in a modern two-story building with groomed roses in front and an enclosed parking lot behind. Upstairs was Administration, quiet and carpeted, with small offices and its own entrance. Downstairs was where the action was. A waiting room for patients took up half the space; the other half, separated by a wall, was where Medicine was—the examining rooms, the laboratory, and the doctors' office, which was just a room with four steel desks. Everything I'd ever learned was useful there. Sometimes I would flash back to the psychiatric locked ward at the VA, or find myself drawing on medical school's long-ago rotations through obstetrics, ophthalmology, and orthopedics, or using what I'd learned in Nepal or the little clinic.

But the Big Clinic was better than all the rest because there was a whole world in its building, and it was social and comradely. There were the gossipy medical assistants, the sour-faced RN who triaged from her cubbyhole, the receptionists, the lab tech. There was the ironic physician assistant and the socialist Dr. Brigit; there was the Colombian family practitioner with the ponytail and thick black mustache who fertilized his orchids, he told me one day with glee, with birth control pills. Almost every day we would go out to lunch together and see our patients—the diabetics drinking Coke, the hypertensives eating nachos—and be served by them, too.

The Big Clinic's patients came from everywhere, the waves of every war leaving its polyglot flotsam on the doorstep. So we saw everything. After the Vietnam War, the Vietnamese arrived, then the Cambodians and the Hmong. Wars in South America brought Guatemalans, Salvadorans, and Nicaraguans. After the revolution in Iran came Persians, and just as I was starting, Afghans were fleeing Afghanistan as the Russians marched in. There were even Sikhs from some political problem I didn't know about. In the exam room, the Sikh men would take off the turban with comb, the steel bangle, the curved knife, and cotton underbreeches that each wore, and place them on the counter, unperturbed that their doctor was a woman. And, of course, there were many patients from Mexico, documented and undocumented.

They would all wait together in the waiting room—children, babies, pregnant women; working men with chest pain, lacerations, and coughs; the middle-aged with back pain, hypertension, and depression; the elderly, the sad, the confused—and everyone had something I could find to like, usually the same thing: they had spirit, they had spunk. They didn't complain, they didn't expect much, and they were grateful.

Mr. Moustique, for instance.

Alette, one of the physician assistants, had asked me to see him. She was worried. "He just doesn't look right," she told me.

And sure enough, I found poor Mr. Moustique sitting in a cockeyed position on the exam table, his head bent to the left, his eyes jiggling to the right.

"Mr. Moustique! What happened?"

"Oh, it was about two weeks ago, I was walking with my son, and suddenly I was thrown to the ground—by what, I don't know—and ever since I have lost my balance."

"Did you pass out?"

"I don't think so, but I cannot drive the car right anymore and my wife, she is scared. She made me come in. I have to put my head like this." He tilted his head even more to the left.

"And drive like this." He pantomimed his head out the car window, "or everything is crossed."

I examined him. He appeared to have "cerebellar syndrome," most likely from a blood vessel that had bled into his cerebellum, which is the part of the brain that controls balance. It's an isolated part of the brain, tucked away, and depending on the cause, can permanently incapacitate the patient with vertigo and loss of balance.

So Mr. Moustique needed to be admitted to a hospital for a workup. Unlike most of our patients, he had health insurance, but even so, it wasn't easy. The County Hospital was full and he had to be admitted to a private hospital, which took me five phone calls. First, I had to talk to the emergency room doctor, who agreed Mr. Moustique should be admitted. Then I had to convince the deputy administrator of his health plan, who had never heard of the cerebellum. Then the admitting physician, the neurologist, and the hospital's administrator. It took me longer to get Mr. Moustique admitted than it had to diagnose him, but eventually it was arranged, he was admitted, and Fast Medicine did a good job. It fixed him.

The biggest change for me from before my residency was that now I was The Internist, and the family practitioners and physician assistants consulted me on complicated cases. And I was at ease, so much so that I could begin to practice medicine not the way I'd been taught but the way I wanted. Which is the advantage of the guild system—once you become a master, you are allowed to do what you think is best.

I did this for the first time with Mrs. Quinones.

Two months before, Alette had discovered that Mrs. Q had diabetes. She started Mrs. Q on insulin, educated her about diet, and taught her to check her own sugars. But she had been unable to get Mrs. Q's sugars, her "blood glucoses," below 400. Normal (nonfasting) is below 140. Consequently, Mrs. Q was still having the symptoms of out-of-control diabetes—blurry vision, frequent urination, thirst, and weakness. So Alette had been increasing Mrs. Q's insulin every week, until now she was injecting herself with 60 units every morning and 40 units every afternoon, but her glucoses were still over 400. Plus she'd gained fifty pounds. Would I take over?

Then Alette introduced me to Mrs. Q, who was short, squat, and 205 pounds. Today we would say she had "metabolic syndrome," but at the time I simply noted that she was obese, diabetic, and hypertensive. And apologetic.

"I am so sorry, Doctora. I am trying to lose weight, but I am so hungry and I keep gaining weight and Miss Alette is so nice. I don't eat anything sweet, nothing! And I check my urines and write them down—here they are; and I am still going to the bathroom all the time, and everything is blurry—Am I going blind? I take care of my daughter's baby, and I am so worried!"

Then she handed me the scraps of paper on which she'd written her glucose checks: 4+ sugars in every urine.

Now, the basic problem in diabetes is a deficiency of the hormone insulin, made by the pancreas. And before the discovery of insulin by Fast Medicine, it was a fatal disease, because the role of insulin is to bring glucose, the body's main energy source, into the cells. There is an alternative energy system but it is much less efficient than glucose. So the untreated diabetic will have two kinds of symptoms. First, because glucose cannot get into the cells, the patient is effectively starving; he loses weight and is weak.

Second, since the glucose cannot enter the cells, it stays in the bloodstream and its level rises. This "hyperglycemia" causes a second set of symptoms: frequent urination as the kidneys try to get rid of the excess glucose, which leads to dehydration and thirst; and blurry vision, as the excess glucose pulls water into the eyes. The discovery of insulin changed diabetes's fatal course. Patients could now inject themselves with the insulin they didn't make, their sugars would come down, their eyes clear, their energy come back, and their weight increase.

I looked through Mrs. Q's chart. Alette was right; Mrs. Q did have diabetes. But she had type 2 diabetes, which differs from type 1 diabetes, which had been the first to be understood. Because type 2 diabetes is not a *complete* lack of insulin but a *relative* lack of insulin. The pancreas of a type 2 diabetic does make some insulin, just not enough.

Otherwise, it has the same two sets of symptoms—weakness and weight loss, and, from the hyperglycemia, frequent urination, thirst, dehydration, and blurry vision. Also, type 2 diabetics have the same response to insulin as type 1 diabetics: the additional insulin lowers their sugars. So their vision clears, their frequent urination and thirst resolves, their weakness improves, and they gain weight.

It is that weight gain in type 2 diabetics that had always bothered me. Because the problem in type 2 diabetes is not an *absolute* insulin deficiency but a *relative* insulin deficiency—usually *relative* to their weight. The problem is often that the type 2 diabetic simply doesn't make enough insulin *for how much he weighs.* But he does make some insulin. This means that there is a weight at which many type 2 diabetics should not need injected insulin. And for those patients who are overweight or obese, who have "metabolic syndrome," we know that losing weight can be the answer. It makes the imbalance between the insulin they do make and their weight better. But losing weight is hard. And the insulin we give makes losing weight even harder, just as it did for Mrs. Q.

So there could be *two* strategies for treating the type 2 diabetic who is also overweight. The first strategy would be to give the patient additional insulin. This is the usual treatment and what Alette did. But because that extra insulin causes the glucose to fall, it often causes the patient to get ravenous, eat more, and gain weight, thus exacerbating the *relative lack of insulin.*

The second strategy would be to *not* give the type 2 overweight diabetic extra insulin. What would happen then? I'd always wondered. In theory, the unusable extra glucose would continue to circulate in the blood at a high level; the kidneys would continue to excrete it, the patient would continue to be thirsty, the eyes would continue to be blurry; he would continue to be weak, and *he would continue to lose weight.* Eventually his weight would reach the level at which his own production of insulin would be enough and his glucoses would normalize on their own.

But we only ever use the first strategy. We give the type 2 diabetic insulin, and this almost always causes weight gain, making the *relative* insulin deficiency worse.

I had always wondered about using that second strategy—weight loss—which is the natural reaction of the type 2 diabetic to their high sugars. And now that I was a Board Certified Internist, a Master, albeit a young one, I could try it out.

I went through the chart to make sure that Mrs. Q didn't have another reason for her high glucoses. Alette had done a great job; she had ruled out sources of infection and other hormonal conditions.

Then I went over what Alette had been doing. She'd been seeing Mrs. Q every week. Mrs. Q's urine glucoses would be 4+, so Alette would increase the insulin dose; Mrs. Q would gain more weight; her sugars would continue to be 4+, and Alette would again increase the insulin dose. Since Mrs. Q continued to have glucoses in the 400s, she also continued to have the symptoms of out-of-control diabetes—frequent urination, thirst, blurry vision, and weakness. Except for one—weight loss.

What we were doing was not simply unsuccessful, it was anti-successful. Because the extra insulin we were giving her was causing Mrs. Q to be hungry, to eat more, to gain weight and, therefore, was making her relative lack of insulin worse.

Since more of the same wasn't working, why not try less of the same? Why not use the body's natural reaction to diabetes, which is weight loss, to treat Mrs. Q's diabetes? She was having the other symptoms of hyperglycemia anyway. If she could keep up with her fluid intake and not get dehydrated, slowly her weight would come into balance with the insulin her own pancreas did produce. Perhaps she would not need any extra insulin.

It was a radical approach but no one was watching.

I explained my strategy to Mrs. Q. and Alette. I was going to take Mrs. Q off her insulin and let her body lose weight as she urinated out that unusable glucose. She would need to drink a lot of water, that was the main thing, and come in every day for the first week and then every week after that so we could make sure she wasn't getting dehydrated. It would take weeks, and she would still be thirsty, her vision would still be blurry, but she wasn't going blind, and as she lost weight her sugars would improve on their own. In the short term, high glucoses, which she was having anyway, wouldn't do her any permanent harm.

"Good. I'm glad," she said, shaking her head. "Going blind, it is so scary."

Mrs. Q lived down the street and she came in every day for the first week, and then every week. She drank a lot of water; her sugars stayed in the 400s, and she continued to have the classic symptoms of diabetes she'd had before. But also the fourth—weight loss.

It took three months. But finally Mrs. Q was down to twenty pounds above her dry weight of 140, and her glucoses were also below 140. Her vision sharpened, her strength returned, and she ended up not needing any insulin. I passed her back to Alette, who kept a close eye on her, because of course if she regained weight, her type 2 diabetes would be back.

So I liked being The Internist in that out-of-the-way clinic. It was interesting, satisfying. And with only eighteen patients a day and taking calls from home, it was a pleasure, after the rigors of residency.

I slept, rested, and recovered, and my joy in life came back.

A year passed. And then Dr. Roark, the medical director, unexpectedly resigned, no one knew why, and the executive director, Mr. Carlos Cardenas, invited me Upstairs. I'd met him only once before, at my initial interview.

As I walked up, I was struck anew by how different Upstairs was from Downstairs. It was carpeted, quiet, and cool. It was not one big companionable space. The office doors were closed and it felt empty, almost abandoned.

But the door to Carlos's office was open, he was sitting at his desk and gestured me in. A picture window looked onto the hills; there was a built-in bookcase and a small refrigerator. His desk was dark wood and on it I saw a Mont Blanc fountain pen, a leather briefcase, and medical journals. He invited me to sit down with a Texan twang and a Mexican cadence.

He would get right to the point, he said. By decree of the State, he had to fill the post of medical director with a doctor, and in his four years at the clinic he'd made a number of mistakes. I would make a good medical director, he thought, looking at me speculatively.

I was taken aback. I didn't yet know what I was supposed to do next but I didn't think it was "medical director." Plus, I liked seeing patients. But I'd never been a medical director before, and Upstairs was quiet and peaceful.

Would he be willing to let me do it part-time? I asked. I would spend the mornings being medical director and the afternoons being The Internist, and we could try it out for a year. How about that?

Carlos's eyes narrowed and he looked at me for a bit. He was holding a pencil in his hand, leaning his cheek on it as he looked at me.

Then he nodded. "That will work."

Upstairs turned out to be very different from Downstairs.

I had my own office with a view of the hills, an in-box and an out-box. It was predictable and pleasant. The Upstairs staff came in late and left early, and only now and then, when a new regulation arrived or at budget time, did it erupt into activity. Most of the medical director's job was going to meetings—board meetings, staff meetings, consortium meetings. The attendees were mainly administrators and the meetings seemed to be not so much meetings to accomplish something as meetings that constituted the job itself. Which was how I met the Head of District Twenty-two, who explained to me what those meetings were really about.

I found myself walking out with him to our cars. It was a hot day on a treeless sidewalk. We started talking. I told him how, from a doctor's perspective, it was bureaucracy that was the problem. It took our time. I gave Mr. Moustique as an example—the five calls I'd had to make to get him admitted to the hospital.

The Head of District Twenty-two shook his head. No. The problem was that health-care providers were going to have to learn to do more with less.

I stopped walking. It was the first time I had ever heard the phrase "health-care provider."

"What?" I asked.

"Hunh?" He stopped walking, too. He turned, and we faced each other.

"What's a health-care provider?" I asked him. "What does that mean?" He was thin and tall and I couldn't see his eyes against the light.

"It's the doctors," he answered. "And the nurses and the hospitals and the clinics—it's whoever provides health care—health-care providers."

I was shocked. "And the patients? The people who are sick, who we take care of? What are they?"

"They're health-care consumers."

"That's ridiculous," I said. "Patients are consumers? Like in a restaurant? They consume healthcare?"

"They're health-care consumers," he insisted. "They choose to spend their money on healthcare; they buy it in the marketplace; they consume healthcare."

My patients went through my mind. The heart attacks, the strokes, the cancers, the mental illness. My patients didn't choose to spend money on healthcare. They didn't have any money to spend and then they got sick. Then they came to the clinic or the hospital and depended on me and mine to get them better.

"If anyone is a consumer," I told him, "it's us, the doctors. We're the ones who consume resources—tissue paper and test tubes, silver and palladium, effort, and energy."

The Head of District Twenty-two stared at me for a second and then resumed walking. "Health-care providers," he repeated. "Doctors are health-care providers and patients are health-care consumers. It's the economic model."

In the meantime, Downstairs in the afternoons, I continued to see patients, which is how I met Ric Molina, and if he was a health-care consumer, he should have been an irate one, because he got a portion that was way too small.

It started one afternoon. I picked up my first chart and went out to the waiting room to get the patient and find out how busy it was. I called, "Ric Molina," and a guy in his late thirties stood up. He was wearing a faded flannel shirt tucked into loose jeans and black thick-soled shoes, and he walked over to me with not quite a limp but with hips swinging around rather than legs swinging out—a sign of lower-extremity weakness.

"Just got out of prison, Doc. My legs hurt and I can't walk right."

We went into the exam room, Ric got up on the table, and I looked at him more closely. His hair was black and curly, his skin sallow, and he had dark circles under his eyes. He looked worn, flattened, without that natural confidence, that ebullience, that keeps the Bad Boys in life.

Then he explained. Selling drugs, three years. About eight months ago his back started to hurt and then his legs didn't feel right, or maybe it started with his legs and then his back started hurting, he couldn't remember, and now his legs were kind of numb and sometimes they twitched.

Just then his left leg did twitch, a jerk, almost a kick.

Like that.

Had he seen a doctor?

"You know prison, Doc. It took months and he saw me right before I got out, and gave me Motrin."

It was his spinal cord almost certainly. Probably some kind of mass was growing inside the narrow cylindrical bone box of the spinal column, which protects the nerves that go from brain to arms and legs, bladder and penis, and that mass was starting to put pressure on the spinal cord and interfere with the conduction of those nerves. Since the process had been going on for months, most likely it was a tumor, a cyst, a polyp, or even an abscess, given his probable use of drugs in prison. So I ordered blood tests and a CT scan, but Ric didn't come back for his results, which were normal.

When he did reappear, ten months later, it was with two canes and a friend, unshaven and not very clean, who helped him stand. Ric's face was yellower and pastier than ten months before, and now he walked hunched over, with his legs splayed out. He had a hard time getting up on the table.

"Ric, what happened?" I asked. "Where've you been? You're worse?"

"Yeah. Sorry about that, Doc. That's why I'm here. Gotta getta job, parole and all, but I'm weak, Doc. My arms are okay, but I can't get up and down steps anymore and now . . ." He stopped.

I waited.

"My . . . urine. It's been starting to . . . leak . . . sometimes." He hung his head.

"What about erections?"

His head came up and he looked almost green.

"Your morning erections, when you get up in the morning?"

He shook his head. No erections.

"Since when?"

"Maybe a week ago."

Then I examined him for the second time. His legs were now completely numb; his lower extremity reflexes were hyperactive, and he was weak from his mid-back down. Everything above the mid-back was normal. So that localized it to his lower back, and whatever it turned out to be, it was an emergency, because once a growing mass starts interfering with the nerves to the bladder and penis, it will shortly cause irreparable damage to the spinal cord. Ric needed a STAT admission to the hospital for diagnosis and treatment, I told him. I had reached the end of what I could do.

"How'm I gonna get there?"

"Do you know anyone with a car?"

"The guy who brought me—but he has to go to work. . . . Well, maybe I could ask him."

I called the ER doctor to let him know Ric was coming; I gave Ric a copy of my evaluation and watched as he hobbled out.

And that, I thought, was that.

I didn't hear back from the ER doctor, though, and that was a change, the first dropped stitch in the fabric of the medicine I knew—that professional courtesy.

"Hi, Dr. S. This is Dr. L—thanks for sending Mr. Molina to us. [You always said this, whether you meant it or not.] . . . Yeah, he's pretty bad, don't know what it is. Neurology is seeing him, and will admit him."

That is what I expected to hear but did not. I didn't know whether Ric made it to the ER or whether his friend said no and he shrugged his shoulders. What I did know was that if he made it to the ER with the symptoms he had, he would be admitted, diagnosed, and treated. It was a neurologic emergency.

So the next afternoon when I saw his name on my schedule, I was surprised. "Ric. What happened? Didn't you get to the ER?"

"I did, Doc. They sent me home. They gave me Motrin and told me to take it easy."

"They didn't admit you?"

"Nah."

"The repeat CT didn't show anything?"

"They didn't do a CT. They did X-rays and said it was my back."

I couldn't believe this. This I could not believe. I'd sent him over with every symptom and sign of an impending spinal cord compression and he'd been sent home.

"Ric, you've got to go back to the ER. You have something going on in your spinal cord and we don't know what it is, and they need to find out what it is before you're completely paralyzed."

I called the ER again, and spoke to a different ER doctor. Ric's friend brought him back and this time he was admitted.

Seven weeks later, therefore, when I saw his name on my schedule, I was relieved. Because for him to be seeing me only seven weeks after his admission, it must have turned out to be something treatable—an abscess or a benign tumor—and this was his follow-up visit. He would be bringing me a report, a note, from the neurologist or neurosurgeon.

But no. He had nothing for me. He hadn't been given any medications or a follow-up visit, and I hadn't been sent anything, either.

So I telephoned the hospital and persuaded someone in Medical Records to read me his discharge summary. His diagnosis was "multiple sclerosis myelopathy," she said, and, no, there was no follow-up.

That didn't seem right to me. I can't tell you why, but it just didn't seem to fit the bill. Call it what you like—intuition, or experience, or having seen Ric over the past ten months—but I didn't believe that MS was what he had. So that Saturday I went over to the medical library to see if I could figure out what he did have. It took a few hours but finally there it was, a report on the newly described disease of tropical spastic paraparesis (TSP). It sounded just like what Ric had. Back pain, progressive leg weakness, hyperactive lower-extremity reflexes, negative workup. The cause was HTLV-1, a virus similar to HIV and spread by IV drugs and unprotected sex. Steroids tended to stabilize or even slow down its progression and sometimes even reverse it.

To make sure, that Monday I tracked down the author of the article and presented Ric's case to him. What did he think? Was it TSP?

It probably was, he told me. Ric should be tested for the antibody. If positive, he should be treated with steroids and told, of course, that it was contagious and spread by needles and sex.

Ric's test was positive, and that was what he had: tropical spastic paraparesis. I prescribed steroids, but I can't tell you how well he did, because I didn't see him again. Perhaps the steroids worked, or more likely, he broke parole and was back in prison getting Motrin for his back pain. In any case, I never got over his not getting admitted to the hospital that first time, when he came in with that potentially devastating symptom. He was my first inkling of the kind of results the New Healthcare—provided and consumed for maximum efficiency—would likely achieve.

Meanwhile, Upstairs I was learning to be a medical director.

There was no one to teach me, so, as I'd do with a puzzling patient, I learned from the past. I opened doors, went through everything I could find in the medical director's desk, and read the old reports, memos, and minutes. I strolled around Upstairs and got to know the staff and then Downstairs to see how it looked from an Upstairs perspective.

At first there was a lot of medical directing to do. The physician assistants were my responsibility, and I had to monitor their care. There was firing and hiring. There were protocols to write, there were the State's ever-new rules, regulations, and programs, and there were the complaints of staff about staff.

Then it began to settle down. And one day, about six months after I started, I came in and there was nothing for me to do. A few minor issues, maybe an hour of work. Upstairs was quiet. I went Downstairs. It was running like clockwork.

I went back Upstairs and sat down in my office. I felt superfluous. And then it occurred to me: maybe that meant I was doing a good job. I remembered Ms. Jane Lloyd. Perhaps for an administrator doing a good job means "nothing left to do." Perhaps that is how you recognize a good administrator, and perhaps that is why the administrative staff is always in a flurry, to escape that uncomfortable feeling I had of being superfluous, of perhaps not being—all that necessary.

I was beginning to understand the inner workings of the clinic, which was not a county clinic but a community clinic, and that turned out to be very different. The county clinics grew out of the medieval monastic tradition of taking care of the sick poor; when the monasteries were closed, the parish in England and the county in America took over that duty. So the county clinic was funded by the county, and controlled by the county. There were regulations, bureaucracy, and oversight.

The community clinic, though, came out of that revolutionary moment of the late 1960s. Aquarian rebels, often physicians, with Mao's *Red Book* in hand, established the community clinic as a free clinic whose fundamental principle was a workers' kingdom in a workers' paradise. The Big Clinic, in particular, had been started in a trailer and its doctors and nurses had originally volunteered their time. No one wore a white coat or a white cap; everyone was called by his first name and everyone was equal—a health-care worker serving the community. The ruling body was the community itself, represented by an elected Board who were also the clinic's patients. And it worked pretty well, as long as it was poor.

But it wasn't poor for long. It worked so well that the State took notice and started funding it. The volunteer doctors and nurses began to be paid, not much but something; the health-care workers also began to be paid, minimum wage; a storefront was rented and the clinic moved in. The Board, however, continued to be solely in charge; the community clinic was, after all, a community clinic.

As the years passed, money continued to flow in, a lot of money for that community. By the time I was ensconced Upstairs, the budget was $1.5 million; there were thirty health-care workers, a medical director, and even an executive director. But the whole shebang was still overseen by an elected board of lay community patients. As I would soon find out, this admirable and idealistic structure had one serious flaw.

By this time, the budget cycle had started, and Carlos informed me that I had to make a budget. I should just copy last year's, he told me, and he would get it to me. He never did, though, but someone did, because one morning there it was, and not only last year's medical director's budget but the budget for the entire clinic, which Carlos had not been keen on me seeing.

I read it through. It was fascinating. I could begin to see how the place was put together from a money perspective. It was like getting the medical records on a puzzling patient, the ah-ha! records, the ones that fill in the missing information and start to resolve the mystery.

This year something new was going on, something that had never happened before: the health-care workers were demanding a raise. They had never yet had a raise, and they made right above minimum wage, $5.46 an hour. That was so little that they qualified for the healthcare they themselves provided. They were asking for a 10 percent raise, to $5.87, which would cost the clinic—in total, for all of them—$30,000 a year. Not much. The clinic had it, I knew, from looking at the budget. And yet, the word was that Carlos would not agree to it.

So one morning when I found the door to his office unusually open and he unusually inside it, I put my head in. "Can I come in? I want to talk about the health-care workers' raise."

I sat down and argued my point. The health-care workers hadn't had a raise in four years. They worked hard, they made very little, and the clinic had the $30,000 a year it would cost.

Carlos listened, smiled a little half-smile, and then shook his head no. I didn't understand his people. With them, *"peón buscando patrón."*

He knew I knew Spanish, but how much?

I understood: Every worker is looking for a boss. "The reverse is also true," I parried.

He raised his eyebrows. I had not disappointed.

Yes, that, too, was true, he acknowledged. The boss needed the worker just as the worker needed the boss—but the worker needed the boss more. The thing was, his people would make a *patrón* out of whoever occupied his position, so he, Carlos, might as well be the *patrón*, and a good *patrón*, beneficent to his friends and his friends' friends; maleficent to his enemies and his friends' enemies. The important thing was that he stay the *patrón*. So,

"No raises. No hires either. Times are bad and the Feds are getting tight. We'll be lucky if we don't have to lay people off."

That made me mad. I knew it wasn't true. Because in my exploring I'd also found the budgets from all three years since Carlos had arrived, and I'd tracked the money. During his tenure, the clinic's budget had risen from $1 million to $1.5 million. Salaries made up only $500,000 of that, and I couldn't figure out exactly where the rest went. There were pages and pages of small sums, and it did seem to add up, but Carlos had a lot of wiggle room. He'd found enough money to raise his own salary so far by 7 percent and was raising it the next year by another 15 percent. He'd tripled his own travel budget to $15,000 while halving the budget for patient travel from $3,000 to $1,500. And there was in fact one new hire, for a union-busting lawyer.

I didn't argue with him, and left the room. But three months later, after the lawyer was hired and the health-care workers did not get their raise, I resigned as medical director. In protest. I didn't enjoy Upstairs anyway. Upstairs was where I saw the evil in the world, and I didn't like it, even though it was a small and petty evil.

I continued Downstairs, though, as The Internist, and kept my mornings free for reading, writing, and thinking. There was some thread connecting Carlos and the budget, the health-care economics of the Head of District Twenty-two, the minimum wage of the health-care workers, and Ric's nearly missed diagnosis. It was political; it was philosophical; it was something I was missing, that we were missing.

But I couldn't find it.

And then came Mrs. Herz and a life-changing book.

The Herzes were unusual for the clinic. They were from Austria, and they were old and healthy. Hans was eighty-three and Hedda was seventy-eight, and they had come to the United States in 1956. "It was just time for us to leave, Doctor," they told me when I asked, and I didn't delve deeper.

Hans was tall with white hair parted on the left, and stood straight with broad shoulders and well-defined muscles. Hedda was more crumpled but lively, with light-blue eyes and white hair, and she, too, was well muscled. In Austria they'd lived in a mountain village, and hiked, swam, and lifted weights, and even now, when they went back to visit, they mountaineered. They had a gym in their garage, Hedda told me; they worked out every day and I should come by and see. On her seventy-second birthday, she'd gone on Jack LaLanne's then popular television show and broke the show's record for push-ups, doing them through the first movement of Beethoven's Sixth Symphony. She was very proud of that and told me every time she came in.

Which was why when Hedda called one morning with an urgent request to see me that day, I was surprised.

"I hurt myself, Doctor. I fell on my knee, I tripped. Hans, as usual, left things on the floor, and I went down. It hurts a lot."

I was busy, with more than a full schedule.

"How much does it hurt?" I asked. "Can you walk on it?"

"Oh, *ja*, I can walk on it."

"Is it swollen? Black and blue? Can you bend it?"

"A little swollen. Not black and blue. I can bend it."

It didn't sound serious, but I'd learned that when a patient calls, it's best to see him or her, regardless of how minor it sounds.

"Okay. Come by in the afternoon. I'll fit you in."

Long about three p.m., when things were at their most hectic, I came out of an examining room and there was Hedda with Hans. She was standing in the hall. No cane or crutch, not even a walking stick. She hadn't been checked in yet.

I went over to say hi, and took a look at her knee. There was a little scrape. It wasn't swollen. It wasn't tender, and it had full range of motion.

"It's fine," I said. "It's minor."

She nodded.

It wasn't an easy trip from her house, I knew. Hans had to get the car and drive the streets and park. That's not easy in your eighties. So I wondered.

"Why did you come in?"

She looked at me, serious.

"I knew it would feel better if you touched it."

"Does it?"

"Yes, it does. It's fine. Thank you."

I cleaned the scrape, put a Band-Aid on it, and she and Hans left.

But as I went about the rest of the day, Hedda stayed in my mind. She was strong, she was tough, and she was nobody's fool. She was proud of her strength and her toughness, and yet she had made the trip just so I would touch her knee. It would feel better if I did, and it did feel better.

What was that about?

I remembered Dr. Fong and his "Victoria, these hands!" and Mr. Danska and those dozen red roses. I thought about the strange deep relationship between doctor and patient. Of what I got from my patients, of what they got from me. That was not ever talked about, neither its diagnostic usefulness nor its therapeutic meaningfulness. And yet it was as if underneath the modern model of the body I had been taught there was something, some other kind of body, with a less defined boundary, a body in which we all participate, a body of energies and connections, of invisible causes with visible effects.

I knew it by experience, but I knew nothing about it. And now that I'd had the time to recover from the residency, now that I was in a place I liked, I began to think about everything the New Healthcare was leaving out of the Medicine I'd learned to love, in the way you love a lover who has very many faults.

I began to use my mornings to explore other medical systems—Chinese medicine, Ayurvedic medicine, homeopathy, naturopathy. I read books, I took classes, I went to seminars. There was much to be said for them, and yet I found their concepts too foreign, too strange, to integrate into my own experiences and thoughts.

And then one afternoon, still thinking about this, I was in the library, in the medical anthropology section, looking at books. Native American medicine, folk medicine, Chinese medicine, *Hildegard of Bingen's Medicine*. Interesting. Who was Hildegard of Bingen?

I took it out. Hildegard of Bingen, I read in its introduction, was a twelfth-century German nun, visionary, composer, and medical practitioner, and she had written a book on her medicine that had just been translated from Latin to German and German to English. And as I stood there and read it, I became more and more intrigued.

Hildegard's medicine was not the eye-of-newt and toe-of-frog medicine I expected from a medieval medical book. It was a real medicine for real patients with real diseases I could recognize, but it was based on a model of the body completely different from my modern medical model. I couldn't quite put my finger on *how* it was different. It seemed a lot like Chinese and Ayurvedic medicine. Why was that? Was Hildegard's medicine what used to be practiced before modern medicine? I wondered.

And had it been left out of modern medicine as too old-fashioned, too medieval? Could it be the missing piece of Western Medicine? The one that explained what I had been seeing all these years that didn't fit?

I checked out the book and took it home to study. Little did I know that I had just discovered the invisible structure, the traditional roots of Slow Medicine.

In the meantime, the health-care workers had not given up the fight for their small raise.

After Carlos refused to put it in the budget, they went to their union, which suggested they meet with Carlos to see if he would change his mind. They did, and he wouldn't. Next they wrote a letter to the Board asking it to overrule Carlos. The Board refused. Then they discovered that the Chair of the Board was a friend of Carlos's and that she and others on the Board were not patients of the clinic as the clinic charter required. So they put together a petition demanding that the Board remove itself and hold new elections.

Most of Downstairs was in the union, and we signed the petition and went to the meeting where it would be presented to the Board. I parked and went Upstairs. The room was packed, with the Board sitting at a long table at the front and us sitting at tables along the sides. The president, whom I'd seen Upstairs in Carlos's office, was fanning herself with an agenda. The Board listened and then voted 5 to 0 against accepting the petition—thank you for your attendance, and now the Board has other things to discuss.

We filed out and when I got back to my car I discovered all four of my tires had been slashed.

There was nothing left to do but have a union meeting. All of us, doctors and nurses included, belonged to the same union, a relic of the community clinic's flattening of hierarchy. Marta the lab assistant offered her home for the meeting.

It was a tiny house with an off-white shag carpet. We talked about what we could do to get the health-care workers their raise.

"We already tried a petition to remove the Board," Dr. Brigit noted.

"Well, what did we expect? Carlos owns the Board—everyone knows that," someone else observed.

"What about going over the Board's head?" asked one of the nurses. "To the Supervisors?"

"They'll never support us. They're management."

"What about the newspapers? The press?"

"Too small. We're too small. Besides, we at least have jobs. In this community, five dollars and forty-six cents sounds pretty good—it's something."

Silence.

"We can't strike. Our patients need us. It wouldn't be ethical to walk outside and picket while they were inside, sick."

"No, we can't strike."

It was silent as everyone thought.

"We have no clout," someone said.

"No, we have no clout," someone else agreed.

And suddenly it occurred to me. I had a vision. Not a Hildegardian vision—not flashing lights and angels descending from the heavens, but a vision nonetheless. What was the clinic? Downstairs was the clinic. There was nothing Upstairs that wiped a single tear or bandaged a single cut. We didn't need Carlos and Upstairs. They needed us. We were the clinic from the beginning, that was why we were Downstairs. Upstairs was built on top of us, and without us, Upstairs had no foundation and would collapse.

"We have all the clout," I spoke out. "True, it would be unethical to strike. But what we could do, since we are the clinic, is move it outside, out of the building. That is, after all, how it started. It will be a statement and an action. We can rent a trailer and park it on the other side of the chain-link fence. We can hang out a sign that says 'The Clinic,' and we can see our patients in it, same as always. We'll set up exam rooms. We'll take our blood pressures, look at our slides, write our notes and orders, diagnose and treat. We'll keep track of the visits. But we won't bill. We'll still care for our patients Downstairs but there will be no money for Upstairs."

A silence fell in Marta's living room.

Everyone could see it.

We were the clinic. We had the power.

The next day around eleven a.m., Carlos appeared at the top of the stairs. He looked like he hadn't slept.

He had an announcement to make, he told us assembled below. He had changed his mind. The health-care workers would get their raise.

Throughout the short speech he was edgy though not ungracious, and for the rest of the day, Downstairs was in an odd silence. Why had Carlos given in?

Later we found out why. He had a spy at our union meeting—Marta the lab assistant, in whose house it was held and in whose big purse on the shag carpet a tape recorder had been spinning. Carlos knew about our plans, and the idea of us moving the clinic outside had shocked him into surrender.

So we never did get to try out my vision, which I regret to this day. I have never forgotten the power of that moment on the off-white shag carpet, as all of us health-care workers realized we had the power to make the changes that needed to occur.

If we would only decide to use it.

A Short Pause to Recapitulate,

OR

The Crack in the Cosmic Egg

I t seemed a good note to leave on.

I was ready to do the next thing. I didn't know what it was, but it would have something to do with Hildegard, and for that I would need a peaceful life without politics. Carlos accepted my resignation with alacrity. He had just the teeniest smile under his stern expression, of victory but also of understanding. He was, after all, not only a smart man but an intelligent man.

And then I had another intermission, a gap, some time away from medical practice to reflect on what I'd seen so far. What I'd known as medicine was changing. It was turning into healthcare, and the more self-assured healthcare sounded, the more uncomfortable I felt.

I'd been taught medicine so well, so thoroughly. True it was sexist, it was racist, it was patriarchal and judgmental. But it was also brilliant, effective, and admirable. There was no question that Dr. Greg,

Dr. Gurushantih, Dr. Meryl, and the others had taught me—had insisted on my learning—something valuable and human.

But now, as I thought about the clinic, and Carlos, and the Head of District Twenty-two, the Herzes and Ric Molina, it was as if I could hear different tunes playing, different themes in some composition whose wholeness no one knew.

There was the tune of Administration, which was the tune of power, of getting control, of making money for yourself. There was the tune of Business—of insurance companies and the service companies springing up to make money from all the new ways of "delivering healthcare." And there was the tune of Science, which was that all knowledge is good, all truth is good, but underneath it and hidden was the ethic of Darwinism—inquire and explore, but also publish and patent.

And all three were realizing they could ally themselves with one another in an Administration-Business-Science Alliance. That is what had led to Ric's nearly disastrous non-diagnosis, which nobody but me would ever know about: Administration demanding the cheapest possible service; Business agreeing to provide it; and Science providing tools to allow that to occur—at least in appearance.

Yet behind those three tunes was another tune. If I were a composer, it would be a medieval tune of dancing in a flowery meadow, with harmonium in the background and flutes above, where relationship is key and the theme is attention, quietness, openness. Behind Administration's tune, Business's tune, and Science's tune, I heard this tune, which we, like Mrs. Herz, all do hear, and even dance to.

The Head of District Twenty-two was more dangerous than Carlos.

Carlos, as time would show, would turn out to be a mere crook and a failed person, or at least a person with deep flaws. He, therefore, could be discounted because he was not implicit to the New Healthcare. All he taught me was that healthcare could be used for personal profit. Afterward he could be tried and found guilty, given a plea bargain or a prison sentence. He didn't teach me something I didn't know.

But the Head of District Twenty-two did. His perspective on medicine floored me at the time and continues to do so to this day, because he is still Head of District Twenty-two and over the decades he has embraced every New Idea for Making Healthcare Cheaper. Taylor's *Principles of Scientific Management* applied to health-care workers, as if we were producing healthcare on an assembly line according to management's protocols. Time clocks, quality-assurance measures, electronic health records, complete quality control—he believes in them all, and he doesn't even profit from them, except inasmuch as healthcare provides him a steady job. He must never have had that conversion experience of getting sick on the way to Damascus and being subject to his own health-care production machine.

Carlos could be dismissed. The Head of District Twenty-two could not.

Ric was an important patient for me not because he had demonstrated yet again the power in medical care of logic or caring. He was important because he demonstrated the results that the Head of District Twenty-two would attain. Getting the Right Diagnosis would never be part of Quality Assurance.

And Mrs. Herz demonstrated the opposite. It was pretty inefficient of her to have Hans drive her over, at their age, to wait in the waiting room, just to have the doctor touch her bruise. But it was effective, and where does that go in the protocol?

That was the question I wanted to answer.

And all the while, Hildegard of Bingen was working on me. She funneled the streams pouring from that jug of Aquarius—alternative medicine, feminism, ecology, spirituality.

Her medicine fit in neatly where I found it, in the medical anthropology section of the library, in the midst of folk medicine, Native American medicine, Chinese and Ayurvedic medicine—perhaps too neatly. As translated, she gave such modern advice—exercise, lose weight, avoid sugar and coffee—which seemed anachronistic; I wasn't sure whether coffee and sugar had even been available in 1140s Germany. Her theory, too, seemed startlingly similar to the theories of Chinese and Ayurvedic medicine. Hers, too, was based on maintaining a balance between hot and cold and wet and dry, and a balance also between corresponding universal elements and bodily humors. I wondered: How was it that she had such a similar way of thinking about the body as the Chinese, as the Indian?

Then there was her life itself. Hildegard brought into question what we were always told: that the Middle Ages were benighted, and if we thought the place of women now was bad—imagine! Yet she ran her own monastery, wrote books of theology in Latin, and acted as a doctor, not only to the nuns in her monastery, but also to children, babies, pregnant women, and men, even impotent men! As a woman, she caught my imagination, and she expressed the spirit of feminism that was distilling at the time.

There was her strange concept of *viriditas*, greenness, which fit so well into the organic food movement, ecology, and our modern green concerns.

And last, there were her visions. In the manuscript from her monastery there were illuminations of them, some even full-page, with colors made of gold and silver, jewels, and plant dyes. They were mesmerizing, as wild and as familiar as dreams. A curly-headed young man smells a flower on a stalk as big as himself. A giant queen holds a crowd of people in her arms. A hideous devil shits onto the world. The Cosmic Egg.

That's how Hildegard described her third vision, where she saw the whole universe as an egg, or an egg-shaped thing. At the center of it was the round earth, looking a lot like how we see it from space; out of the earth came the rivers of Paradise. Then around the earth was a dark-blue sky filled with golden stars, and around the blue sky were red-gold flames. At each corner was one of the four directional winds—the North Wind, South Wind, East Wind, and West Wind—painted as faces, blowing. So it was a mandala illustrating the medieval conception of a geocentric universe, with the Winds as the motive power, blowing the sky around the earth. Above the earth, so at the top of the painting, were the medieval planets—Mercury, Mars, Venus, Saturn, Jupiter, and Sun—and below the earth was the sickle moon.

So in one sense Hildegard's vision could be read as a hidden natal astrological chart, showing the very moment when God creates the sun, moon, and planets all at once in the east, sets the winds to blow, and so begins time.

But how was it an egg? I wondered. Hildegard called it an "egg" (in Latin, *ovum*), and in the illumination it *was* an egg, in the sense that it was egg-shaped—an oval—but there was no shell and no yolk. And as I tried to see how it might be an egg, suddenly I realized what the illumination *also* was, and why it was so familiar and so fascinating. I'd seen it many times as I stood at the foot of a bed and waited for a baby's head to crown, and had seen it for the first time, so long ago, when Meg gave birth.

Hildegard's vision of the whole universe, I realized to my shock, was a well-observed, anatomically correct image of birth! The earth at the center was not only the earth but also a vagina; in place of the baby's head crowning were the rivers of paradise. On the outside, the red and gold flames were also the labia majora and minora, and the stars were Bartholin's glands. Below the vagina, the moon was the anus; above the vagina, the planets were urethra and clitoris. It was as true to life as any drawing in my medical books.

It was crazy.

Later I would discover it wasn't as crazy as I'd thought: images of birth were often placed in medieval churches and even had a name— they were called sheela-na-gigs.

But Hildegard's vision was even more profound because in visualizing the Creation as a birth, she'd made a kind of conceptual cat's cradle: out of the body, which is the universe, comes the universe itself. She'd visually answered the question about which comes first, the chicken or the egg.

For Hildegard, the universe was the egg, inside of which was the bodily universe that contained all eggs and all Creation. It was an egg giving birth to itself, and a Jungian mandala of outside and inside uniting. In it Hildegard united those two first images I myself had, so long ago, at the home of my friends the Neumanns, of the whole starry cosmos moving over my head when I lived on that roof, and Meg's birthing in my ex-bedroom. You can't get more poetic than that.

Who was this woman who created, imagined, and presented us with a medieval medical universe of the wholeness of things?

Now I knew what I would do next. I would understand Hildegard's world, and I would start by learning Latin so I could read her close up, in her own language, and not through translations. But to do that I would need to find a different kind of place to work. An un-tire-slashing, un-board-meeting, un-political kind of place where I could concentrate and think in peace.

I would spend the next few months going on interviews, trying to find that perfect position. The last interview would be in a most unlikely setting, a hospital that would turn out to be more perfect than I could ever have imagined. It would not be simply a place away from politics but a place that would demonstrate what Hildegard had to teach.

It would be a Kingdom of Slow Medicine.

FOURTEEN

The Force That Through the Green Fuse Drives the Flower

I drove over for my interview, and when I saw the hospital for the first time, high on a hill overlooking the ocean, I was taken aback. Although I'd had patients admitted to Laguna Honda Hospital in San Francisco before, I'd never visited, and I had imagined it to be some kind of warehouse for the chronically ill. Instead, it looked like a medieval monastery, with cream-colored walls, a red-tiled roof, a bell tower, and turrets.

The medical director, Dr. Major, interviewed me in her office, and then she took me out for the tour.

Originally, she explained as we walked around, the hospital had been San Francisco's almshouse, which was how we used to take care of the sick poor before there was health insurance. There was the County Hospital for the acutely ill, and the county almshouse for everyone else—the chronically ill, those who needed more care before they went home, the unemployed, the homeless, the elderly, the lunatic, orphans—anyone you didn't know what else to do with you could always send to the almshouse. So, typically, it was immense—Laguna Honda sat on sixty-two acres, with 1,178 patients, 32 doctors, 1,500 other staff, a live-in priest, and a resident nun.

It was an ancient model of care, she explained, and went all the way back to the Middle Ages, when monks and nuns took care of the sick poor for free, as part of their vocation. Originally such places were called "God's Hotels," and in France, they still were known as *hôtels-Dieu*. At one time, almost every county in the country had had both a free county hospital and a free county almshouse, but in the 1950s many of the county hospitals and almost all the almshouses were closed, for reasons of justice from the left and economy from the right. Laguna Honda Hospital, she thought, was probably the last almshouse in the country.

Then we walked under a painted statue of Saint Francis, and I saw the long, open Nightingale wards where the patients stayed. We went upstairs and she showed me the X-ray machine where I could read my own films, and the laboratory with a microscope where I could make my own slides. We walked past a 1950s-era beauty salon with steel-helmet hair dryers, and I saw the chapel, which was more like a small church, really, with stained-glass windows, polished wooden pews, and a very politically incorrect Stations of the Cross along the walls. We went outside and she showed me the greenhouse, the aviary, and the little farm, so that patients could pot plants, watch chickens hatch from eggs, and see animals, even if they were bedbound. Then we walked back to her office and she offered me the job.

I didn't know. I wasn't sure. That hospital was like no hospital I'd ever seen or even imagined. But with no call and no weekends, it was the only place I'd found where I would be able to both practice medicine and also study Hildegard. So I hedged my bets. I told Dr. Major I would come temporarily, for two months. I didn't think she would accept.

That was fine with her, she said. She needed another doctor on the Admitting Ward.

The Admitting Ward?

That was where every patient first came. Like the other wards, it had space for thirty-six patients, and there were three doctors for the three new admissions every day. Although it was fast-paced, sometimes hectic, I would have plenty of time to examine my patients, work them up properly, and follow them. I would like it.

I did like it.

It would be the most fascinating place I'd ever practiced, and I wouldn't leave after two months. Partly because, as an almshouse, it took care of the bottom one-tenth of 1 percent of the City's population of 550,000, and its patients, therefore, were three standard deviations from the mean. Any mean. They were the tallest and shortest, the fattest and thinnest, the best and worst patients I'd ever had, and they had almost every disease, too. So I learned a tremendous amount of medicine there. Almost every disease in *Harrison's* showed up, because if a disease occurred in one in a hundred thousand patients, we would see at least one.

The three patients we admitted every day usually arrived in the late morning from the County Hospital, from private hospitals, from their homes if they had them, or sometimes directly from the streets. So I had most of the morning to organize my other eleven patients, who would be at various stages of recovery. I would stroll around the ward and take a look at each of them, talk to the nurses, go over their labs, run upstairs and check on their X-rays from the day before, and then I would write my orders. It was a lot like being an intern but less stressful. By the time my admission arrived, my other patients would be organized, and I would have most of the day, barring emergencies, to work up my new patient.

I soon learned that the most important thing was to see my new patient as soon as he arrived, even before looking at the records or talking with the family. It wasn't how I'd been taught, but that way I could reach my own conclusions, uncontaminated by any preexisting diagnoses. So as soon as the new patient was in bed, I would walk down the ward, find him, sit on his bed or in a chair, and we would just look at each other for that first minute, which is the beginning of a long-term relationship. Everything that will ever come up is already there, if you only knew. I would see how clean or dirty he was, how happy or sad, scared, fretful, or at peace. I would get an immediate sense of how sick he was, and of how much life force I had to work with, which is the most important measure of all.

We would talk, but not much. We would talk later. I would examine the patient first.

Because, although today there is a movement to discredit or even ban the physical examination as not "evidence based," not "objective," there is nothing better, more informative, than thoroughly examining a patient. Not as a ritual, not because it is traditional, not in order to strengthen the doctor-patient relationship, but simply because the body is where the diagnoses are. Dr. Gurushantih had convinced me forever.

Only after that would I go back to the doctors' office and go through the records, page by page. There were always discrepancies, discordant diagnoses, multiple medications for the same problem. Then I would talk with the family, call up the previous physicians, try to resolve the discrepancies and establish the real diagnoses. I would order them from most important to least important, the way Dr. Dan Kelly had taught me so long ago. Finally, I would write up the story of the patient using the elegant format of modern medicine: history, physical exam, labs and X-rays, assessment, and plan.

Day by day I would work through that plan, reformulating it as things became clear. Since the new patient would usually stay on the Admitting Ward for weeks, I had the time to straighten things out, to make sure that when he did leave, he had the right diagnoses and the right treatments.

Not only did I have the time to get the right diagnoses and the right treatments, but so did the nurses. So when the patient left, he or she was also buffed and polished—beard shaved or hair styled, nails trimmed, wounds on their way to healing. The social workers had enough time too, as did the therapists—everyone had enough time to do their work well. And although on paper all that time might have seemed inefficient, I was continually impressed by how efficient it was, even from a health-care economist's point of view.

For example: Patients would typically come in on between fifteen and twenty-six medications, of which they actually needed only four or five. They would have accreted all those medications over the years, as their doctors, not having the time to discontinue a perhaps unnecessary medication in a stable patient, would simply renew everything. They would have gathered diagnoses, too, serious diagnoses they didn't actually have, or had no longer—seizures, diabetes, hypertension, even cancer or AIDS—for which they were taking medications and getting lab tests. Establishing the correct diagnoses, and then getting them off all those unnecessary medications, with their side effects and adverse reactions, took a lot of time, but in the long run it saved way more money than it cost. It was slower but it was better.

I saw this again and again but I didn't have a way to think about it until the Slow Food Movement finally arrived on our shores. As it did and I began to understand it, I could see that it had intriguing resonances with the medicine I'd been learning over so many years.

Slow Food was not really about fast or slow in time. Rather it was about privileging the basics—the ingredients, which do take time: farmers' time and gardeners' time, and also their skill, experience, and knowledge. It was about accepting what is—the seasons, weather, climate—and flowing with it, not against it. It was about removing what is in the way of a plant being the healthiest, the most fertile, the happiest it could be, and doing so by little actions, by fussing and fiddling. That was how it was "slow."

Slow Food was about process, I gradually understood. Even with the best ingredients you can't have a good meal if all you focus on is the product, the result. So it meant a certain Way, a certain style of preparation. Sipping a glass of wine as you prepare the food, tasting what you are making along the way, not necessarily following a recipe exactly, because—how can you? This tomato and that potato have terroir, were grown differently from any other tomato and potato, had different amounts of flavors, of sweet, sour, earthy, piquant. So each dish was individual, one of a kind, and couldn't be replicated according to algorithm or protocol. The same recipe would give a different flavor, taste, and texture, every time.

Slow Food was local, individual, and relational.

And like the medicine I was doing on the Admitting Ward, Slow Food wasn't more expensive than Fast Food, either, though it seemed as if it should be. It was less expensive, as my friend Rosalind would prove a few years later, when she took the food-stamp challenge of trying to feed her family on a food-stamp budget. She lost weight and filled up two freezers in the process. She spent more time but she saved money.

Slow Food began to infuse itself into my way of thinking. But the connection between it and medicine only began to gel for me after my patient Mrs. Persily, and what happened when I didn't treat her.

Until Mrs. Persily, I thought it was ironic—rule number thirteen of Samuel Shem's *The House of God*, the novel of internship whose irony I took as my guide.

I had tried its other rules. Rule number three: "At a cardiac arrest, the first procedure is to take your own pulse." Rule number twelve: "If the radiology resident and the medical student both see a lesion on the chest X ray, there can be no lesion there." But I had never tested rule number thirteen: "The delivery of medical care is to do as much nothing as possible."

There was a reason for that. By then, I believed in medicine. I'd been convinced. Surgery worked, anesthesia worked, antibiotics and IVs, EKGs, lab tests, and X-rays worked. They put to sleep, removed cancers, cured infections, diagnosed heart attacks. All my doctor friends believed in medicine, too. So we treated everything as we'd learned to do in medical school, internship, and residency.

What occurred this particular month, however, was that Dr. Major closed the Admitting Ward temporarily, in order to make her point about what would happen if a budget cut to the hospital was not rescinded. For the meantime, I'd been assigned to Ward L8, a ward of the terminally demented women, whose head nurse was Mrs. Blake, from Liberia.

Mrs. Blake was slim, small, neat, and pretty, with a brown-black, lineless countenance, a straight nose, firm jaw, and compressed lips. She was pro-life at both ends of the spectrum, I had heard, and she was devoted to the continuing existence of each of her thirty-six charges, no matter what it took, and regardless of the fact that most of them were mute and contracted, giving signs of life only when blood was drawn or a feeding tube inserted.

On my first morning on Ward L8, Mrs. Blake handed me the stack of monthly orders I was to sign. I sat down at the nursing station, started to go through them, and gradually realized that at the end of almost every one was an order for a feeding tube.

Feeding tubes are little rubber tubes that can be inserted through the nose down the esophagus into the stomach if artificial nutrition is necessary. They were first used in the 1950s by surgeons so that surgical patients temporarily unable to eat could continue to get the calories, proteins, and vitamins they needed to recover from their surgery. In the 1960s, the tubes spread to medicine, and they began to be used to feed those who were permanently unable to eat, usually from a catastrophic stroke or as the final common pathway of end-stage dementia. There are two problems with them. First, patients hate them and demented patients try to pull them out, and therefore have to be restrained, that is, tied to the bedposts, to prevent this. Second, once a feeding tube is placed, a patient can be kept alive almost indefinitely.

Most people, when asked, say they don't want a feeding tube to keep them alive if they are terminally ill, although some do. So as I went through the orders and Mrs. Blake stood impatiently behind me, I was trying to figure out: Did these patients want to be kept alive with these tubes? Had they agreed to them? Had someone?

Who had consented to all these feeding tubes? I asked Mrs. Blake.

She frowned. No one had to consent. It was feeding. The patients who didn't eat any longer had to be fed with a tube. If they weren't fed, they would die.

"But you want me to sign an order for them. Do the families agree to them?"

Mrs. Blake did not answer.

I left the stack of orders and went over to Dr. Major's office to discuss with her what I should do.

Unless someone wanted to be kept alive with a feeding tube, I told her, I didn't think they should be, and there wasn't any evidence that any of these patients wanted to be. At the end of life, it was natural to stop eating and drinking. After a certain point, patients simply turned their heads when the nurses put a spoon to their lips. If the nurses tried to force-feed them, they coughed, and if they had a feeding tube, they had to be restrained or they pulled it out. They still got aspiration pneumonias, in spite of the tubes, even though the idea was that the feeding tube would prevent aspiration as well as provide nourishment. Did I have to sign those orders? Didn't the patient or the family have the right to be told, to be asked, and even to refuse?

Dr. Major knew all about Mrs. Blake and her feeding tubes, she told me. They were a problem throughout the hospital. We'd never made a concerted effort to find out from patients what they wanted at the end of life. So she had formed an ethics committee to look into that; would

I like to be part of it? It would take a while to organize, however, and in the meantime, I should choose my battles wisely.

I would like to be on the committee, I told her.

And then I returned to Mrs. Blake, sat down, and signed the stack of orders.

Ward L8 was amazingly peaceful. It seemed that once a patient was that demented, she reached some new strange plateau of stability. It was a kind of Newtonian First Law of Living: Life continues until something gets in its way. Very little happened. No one got sick. All thirty-six hearts continued to beat, all seventy-two lungs to inhale, all thirty-six brains to process whatever minimum was needed for those two activities, and what else was there to fail?

But then on Monday morning of my last week, Mrs. Persily turned up ill.

I came in that morning, and Mrs. Blake informed me that Bed Number 24, Mrs. Persily, had a fever of 104, she was coughing, and her blood pressure was low. I would have to transfer her to the Acute Ward so she could get antibiotics, oxygen, and IVs for her pneumonia. Then she handed me the doctor's order for the transfer, already written by herself. All I had to do was sign it.

"Is that what her family wants us to do?" I asked.

"She has pneumonia. She has to go to the Acute Ward. We can't treat her here, she'll die."

"I think I'll take a look at Mrs. Persily first," I told her.

Then I walked down the long ward—ladies to left of me, ladies to right of me, ladies in front of me, curled up and contracted, with yellow bags of tube feeding by most of the beds, drip-dripping.

I found Mrs. Persily lying curled up on her right side. There wasn't much left of her. Not much fat on her body, not much frizzled hair on her head, not much movement except for her eyes, which were open, roving back and forth, seeing nothing. She was very hot, her pulse was rapid, and her breathing was shallow—almost certainly she had pneumonia.

I remembered what Dr. William Osler, the great physician of the beginning of the twentieth century, had called pneumonia. He had called it "the old man's friend," because in those pre-antibiotic days, it took the patient so rapidly. I thought about Mrs. Blake's order for me to sign, which would send Mrs. Persily to the Acute Ward, where her pneumonia would be cured in a week. I would be taking the possibility of that quick and easy death away from her, saving her for the progression of her dementia, an eventual feeding tube, restraints, and a prolonged dying. I remembered Mrs. Carmona.

I returned to the nursing station, got her chart, and telephoned the daughter listed on the admitting sheet. I explained the situation and asked her: Should we transfer her mother to the Acute Ward to treat her pneumonia?

What else can we do? the daughter asked. I thought we had to treat her pneumonia.

Well, no. We could keep her here, keep her comfortable, and let Nature takes its course. What would her mother want us to do, if she could tell us?

We never talked about it, she said.

She was quiet for a few moments. Then, Let's do that, she said. That sounds right; I'm sure that's what Mother would want. Let's keep her on the ward. Would I call her sister and explain? And their brother?

Sure.

It took me an hour to make those calls, but by the end, the family was in agreement. Their mother would stay on the ward without antibiotics, oxygen, or IV, and we would let Nature takes its course.

Mrs. Blake was outraged, and after I left, she called back the two daughters and the brother and tried to argue them out of Nature. But they held fast.

The next morning, as I was walking over to the ward, I thought about Mrs. Persily. She would be much worse—her temperature higher, her breathing more labored, with a weak cough. Perhaps I should prescribe narcotics, which would help with the dyspnea, the shortness of breath, that dying of pneumonia can cause.

When I got there, however, and walked over to see her, I was surprised. She was lying in bed, breathing comfortably. I felt her forehead. Her fever was down. I took her pulse. It was slower and her respirations were fewer. She seemed slightly better. And that was the last thing I'd expected.

All day long I waited for the call that she had died. It never came. Instead, when I went back to check on her before I went home, she was even better, and by the next morning, she was back to her usual state of health. The nurse was feeding her breakfast, she was sitting up in bed, opening her baby-bird mouth and swallowing whatever was spooned in. She had no fever and no cough. There was no doubt about it—Mrs. Persily's pneumonia was cured, or perhaps *healed* would be the better word to use.

I was stunned. It wasn't as if Mrs. Persily was young. If pneumonia could kill anyone, it should have killed her. And yet there she was with no fever, a normal pulse, and normal respirations. Had she been transferred to the Acute Ward and received its oxygen, antibiotics, and IVs and improved in the same way, I would have thought it just one more piece of evidence of the power of modern medicine. And yet Mrs. Persily hadn't received anything. And her pneumonia was gone.

Something else had cured it, and that could only be Nature, which, after all, we had let take its course.

Then I thought again of Dr. William Osler. This time I remembered his statistics. Before antibiotics, 25 percent of patients with pneumonia died. So—a lot. But that meant that 75 percent of patients with pneumonia did not die. Which meant that Nature cured them. That's quite a lot of curing, when you think about it. If Nature were a medicine, she would be patented and sold for quite a bit of money.

By this time I knew from my study of Hildegard and the premodern medicine she represented that our ancestors had known about this healing power of Nature. They even had a name for it—the *vis medicatrix naturae*. "Nature" from the Latin *natus*, from *nasci*—to be born—so "Nature" is what you are born with, who you are. In Greek, "Nature" is rendered as *physis*, which is the root of *physician*, and which comes from the verb *phuein*—how a plant grows.

None of us is a stranger to *physis*—we all know that plants grow, produce flowers and fruits, die, and then grow back again. We even know human *physis*. We see it all the time—the cut that heals, the cold that goes away, the bruise that resolves, the fracture that even modern medicine can only set to heal on its own. But we never think about it. I didn't, until Mrs. Persily.

But after Mrs. Persily, I did think about it. I began to wonder how many of the cures I'd seen during my life as a doctor were not from the miracles of modern medicine but even, perhaps, in spite of them. And I began to ponder not only what I could do for my patient but what I could *not* do for him, how I could get out of the way of Nature.

By the time Mrs. Persily had fully recovered, it was the end of that month, and Dr. Major had won her budget battle. What had happened was that after she closed the Admitting Ward, the County Hospital had no place to send its not-yet-completely-healed patients, and so it filled up, and then had to close its doors to new admissions. The private hospitals then had to accept the county's uninsured, unreimbursable sick poor, which was terrible for their bottom lines, and they put as much pressure as they could on the Board of Supervisors, which rescinded our budget cuts.

Dr. Major reopened the Admitting Ward, and I happily returned to it.

Meanwhile, I had decided to go back to school and get a PhD in medical history with Hildegard of Bingen as my focus.

My idea was to understand Hildegard and her medicine from the inside, by learning her language, her culture, and her history as she knew it. Or, better, as her student would have known it. So during the days when I wasn't at the hospital and taking care of patients, I began taking classes in medieval Latin and German, paleography, medieval history, medical anthropology, and folklore. Soon I was able to read what Hildegard wrote in Latin, and for comparison I tracked down and read every contemporary twelfth-century medical text I could find.

I also began to experiment, the way I imagined her student might have done. I grew her medicinal plants in my garden, I cooked up her potions and syrups, I brewed her medicinal beers and baked her antidepressant cookies. And slowly I began to understand how Hildegard's model of the body differed from my own modern, mechanical model of the body, and why it was so similar to the Chinese model and the Ayurvedic model of the body. It was because it came out of her experience, and the general premodern experience, of a rural agricultural world—out of her experience, that is to say, as a gardener, as an herbalist.

Our modern idea of the body is that the body is a machine or a collection of machines. So the brain is a computer, the heart a pump, the kidney a filtering device. Even the cells that make up the body we imagine as machines. The cell is a factory, its mitochondria a powerhouse, its nucleus a computer with DNA as its code. In this model, disease is a mechanical breakdown, and the doctor is a mechanic whose job is to find what is broken and repair it or replace it. We can't help it. We are surrounded by machines and we naturally understand the hidden, invisible inner body through the ideas and metaphors around us.

Hildegard lived in a world much more like the world of Nepal. It was a green world, the world of the farmer, of the gardener, of seasons, of weather, of plants. And that mattered, because even though Hildegard was a mystic, theologian, composer, and visionary, she had also been the *infirmarian*—the medical practitioner—for her monastery, and so down-to-earth, literally. Every monastery had an infirmarian who was responsible for the medical care of the monks or nuns, the monastery workers and their families, and anyone who knocked on the door—travelers, visitors, the sick poor. It was a vocation, and it entailed not only caring for the sick but also preparing their herbal medications. As infirmarian, Hildegard was also her own herbalist; she herself grew and prepared the medicines she used as medical practitioner.

Consequently she lived in two overlapping worlds—the world of her garden and the world of the body—and she took the concepts and style that worked in the garden—fussing and fiddling, process, and slowness—from her plants to her patients. That is, she interpreted what she saw in her sick patients with what she knew from her garden about the well-being of her plants. And she did so, I discovered, through her idiosyncratic use of the particular Latin concept of *viriditas*.

Viriditas comes from the Latin for "green," *viridis*, and means "the state of being green," so "greenness." It was a well-researched concept already in Hildegard's theology. Scholars of her work interpreted it as meaning the divine force of life, the shining presence of God—as an abstraction, really, a notion.

But as I studied her medical writings, I discovered that in medicine Hildegard did not use *viriditas* to mean something abstract but something physical. Every plant has its own *viriditas*, she wrote, its own specific medicinal essence. And when we eat a particular food, the *viriditas* of that food comes into the body and changes its *viriditas*. *Viriditas* as a concept was a kind of final common pathway for all the effects of outside on inside, and I wondered whether it was unique to Hildegard, or not.

So I spent a year following the tracks of *viriditas*. It led me backward through the Arabic translations of Greek medical and horticultural texts, to the first known horticultural treatise in the West, by Theo-phrastus. There I found the Greek equivalent of Hildegard's *viriditas*, and there it meant specifically the "green sap of plants." There, too, it was the final common pathway for all the external influences that acted on a plant—weather, climate, and terroir.

Hildegard did, however, do something unique with this originally horticultural concept, she applied it to the human body. Human beings had their own *viriditas*, she assumed, and in the body it was both a power, that healing power of Nature I'd seen in Mrs. Persily, and a sub-stance, which was the final common pathway, in human beings as in plants, for all external influences: weather, climate, and the seasons, food and drink, activity and rest, temperament, attitude, and sex.

Thus arose Hildegard's implicit idea, which for me was revolutionary, that as a doctor I should be not only a mechanic of the body, looking for what is broken and trying to fix it, but also a gardener of the body, nourishing *viriditas*, and removing what is in its way.

After I finally understood Hildegard's *viriditas*, I found myself not only looking at my patient with the eye of a modern doctor—asking myself, What's wrong? And how can I fix it?—but also stepping back and looking at my patient in the context of his environment, and asking myself: What can I do to remove what's in the way of *viriditas*? And what can I do to fortify it?

I would still go out and see my patient cold, without looking at his records, still sit with him, examine him, and then go over all his records and talk with the family. I would still use the brilliant method I'd been taught in medical school. I would still, that is to say, lead with Fast Medicine, with the model of body as machine and doctor as mechanic, and ask myself, What is wrong? And how can I fix it?

But I would also, at the same time, while I was being the mechanic and practicing Fast Medicine, somewhere in the back of my mind be practicing Slow Medicine. I would also think like a gardener and see the body as a plant. And ask myself, therefore, How is this patient doing, globally, as a whole? Is he thriving? Or shriveling? I would watch and feel and estimate the patient's life force, his healing power of Nature, his *viriditas*. And I would ask myself, What is interfering with this patient's life force? What is in the way of him thriving?

To find out, I would put the patient back in the context of his environment, I would visualize him within his environment—body, skin, bedclothes, ward, city, life—like a camera zooming out. I would think about what he was eating, drinking, taking in, literally and figuratively. Were there medications I could discontinue, was there discomfort I could assuage, pain I could treat, anxiety I could allay? What could I do to remove those things or palliate them?

And last, what could I do to fortify his *viriditas*? Change his diet? Get him a beer or a cup of tea? New clothes? Company?

I found myself practicing a kind of Fast Medicine and Slow Medicine together—at many different levels. At the level of actual time, of course, but even more, at the level of style. Mechanic *and* gardener. Focused *and* diffuse. The parts *and* the whole.

And then I began to realize that something strange was going on. Something disconcerting.

After I'd done all that, learned all that, figured out all that—what was wrong with the patient and what wasn't wrong with him, removed as best I could what was in the Way, fortified *viriditas*, turned down the dripping of the tap of life, done everything I could think of to do, then, suddenly—there we were. The patient, who seemed, after our long acquaintance, just another person like myself. There he was, in his predicament, and me in mine. He knew me about as well as I knew him: my flaws and weaknesses, my virtues and strengths; when I would "just sit" with him, he was also just sitting with me.

There we both were. Waiting for Godot.

And I did less and less with my patients, and they got better and better.

FIFTEEN

Nothing Is Better Than Life

A nd then things started to change.

It began during the years I was working on my PhD and realizing just how efficient Slow Medicine was. What happened was that the hospital was discovered. First by the health-care efficiency experts and then by the lawyers of the Department of Justice, and neither liked what they found. The greenhouse! The aviary! The little farm! The live-in priest! The resident nun! But especially the big open wards. They didn't like those at all. The hospital was violating its patients' civil right to privacy, the Department of Justice decided, and the City would have to either rebuild it as a modern healthcare and rehabilitation facility or shut it down.

A lot of battles and politics followed. Letters to the newspapers. Meetings and protests. Hirings and firings. It became harder and harder to practice medicine there. Yet I was determined to stay. Because the City did pass a huge bond to replace the old hospital with a shiny new Facility for the Providing of Health Care, and I wanted to see how it would all turn out, whether the old hospital's style could weather such a change in venue. And this was how I would meet Mr. Nicks and learn how to be slow in the midst of fast, and fast in the midst of slow.

In preparation for the move to the new health-care facility, the Admitting Ward was permanently closed, and in its place I was assigned to Dr. Bee's ward. She met me on my first morning there and we walked around the ward together, from Bed Number 1 to Bed Number 32, the number of beds having been decreased from thirty-six to thirty-two in a futile attempt to placate the Department of Justice. Dr. Bee told me about each patient and introduced me to them.

I had never seen such a collection.

They were in their thirties, forties, and fifties, and almost all were "triple diagnosis" or even "quadruple diagnosis" patients, with a medical, psychiatric, and social diagnosis. So each had the rare disease that had brought him to the hospital; each also had a psychiatric diagnosis—schizophrenia, manic-depression, psychosis nonspecified—and often also a character disorder—narcissism, borderline, obsessive-compulsive. The third, "social," diagnosis was drug abuse—heroin, cocaine, alcohol, and marijuana.

In the past, these patients had been scattered throughout the hospital on different wards in order to even out the load, because each required so much doctor and nurse time. But then, in accordance with a new progressive nursing theory, they had been relocated to a single ward so that staff could become expert at their kind of care. Immediately afterward, however, the economy tanked and with it the hospital's budget. As a cost-saving measure, pay was cut, and the most experienced staff were retiring as fast as they could. The result was that the most difficult patients were all in one place, and there were fewer and fewer experienced staff to take care of them.

We reached Bed Number 19, and Dr. Bee began to tell me about its patient, Mr. Raymond Nicks. He was fifty-two. His drug abuse spanned the spectrum—heroin, cocaine, marijuana, and alcohol. His psychiatric disorder was "schizoaffective," which meant he was not only schizophrenic but also depressed. His rare disease was "bilateral thalamic stroke," which was so rare that Mr. Nicks was my first and only.

There's a reason for its rarity. The thalamus, in Greek *thalamos*—"an inner or secret chamber"—is a knot of tissue beneath the cerebrum. So it lies between the big brain and the rest of the body, and it is the brain's hub, switchboard, CPU—whatever metaphor you want to use, from whichever century. Almost all messages, from above or below, pass through it, and it modulates them, connects them, and sends them on. Like most of the brain, the thalamus has a left side and a right side. Each side is responsible for somewhat different functions, but each can also compensate, to a certain extent, for the other. So a stroke on one side of the thalamus is devastating but survivable. Having strokes on both sides of the thalamus, however—a "bilateral thalamic stroke"—is nearly always fatal.

But Mr. Nicks had somehow, with the tenacity, the good bad luck and the bad good luck of our patients, survived. And he had the terrible scars to show for it, I saw, as I stood in front of him and Dr. Bee talked.

He was a light-colored African American, husky, with a square face, wide forehead, splayed nose, and warm brown eyes. His graying hair was close-cropped and nappy, and he had a thick, rectangular, salt-and-pepper mustache over full lips. He looked a lot like those Egyptian statues of the early pharaohs, with their square faces, short hair, and mustaches. Later when I got to know him, it was easier to see how handsome he must have been in his prime. A real dandy and irascible, his sister would tell me.

But the devastation of those bilateral thalamic strokes was what stood out. His right eye looked at us, his left eye went outward and askew. He couldn't use his hands to feed himself, their movements were so unmodulated. He couldn't walk. He could sit in his wheelchair—dressed, fed, and shaved by the nurses—and he could look at us attentively, but he could not listen because, as Dr. Bee went on to tell me, Mr. Nicks was also deaf, apparently from a bout of meningitis as an adolescent. Nor could he speak. When he tried, he had the speech of the deaf, but perhaps that was from the thalamic strokes. He was, nevertheless, able to read and write.

He was?

Yes, Dr. Bee said. It took him a long time, but if you wanted to communicate with him, he could read your questions and write his own answers, in longhand. Writing on a clipboard seemed to stabilize his movements. That's how she'd obtained his "living will"—his Advanced Life Directives. It had taken her an hour, but you just had to be patient.

What were they?

Oh, he wanted everything done. Everything to keep him alive.

Anything else I should know?

Nothing much. His seizures were well controlled. Agitation, depression, maybe schizophrenia, also well controlled. Drug abuse not a problem. Nice, involved sister. He was a sweetie.

Dr. Bee's ex-ward turned out to be the hardest ward I ever had, and the time, the hardest at the hospital.

The economy continued to collapse, and our budget continued to be cut, with doctors, nurses, and social workers being laid off in waves. The hospital was preparing to move from its comfortable, decrepit, monastic-style digs into shiny, modern, computer-controlled buildings. The Department of Justice had been joined in its crusade by the Health Care Financing Administration, and by a convocation of disability lawyers, and all were pursuing any signs of weakness from the City. Administration decided, therefore, that the forms, regulations, committees, and meetings that all these investigations required should take precedence over patient care. Which sounds terrible but had a kernel of truth. Any one of those investigating magistrates could close the hospital down, or at the least, ensnare it so badly that it would go down of its own accord.

At the same time, my new patients were the sickest patients I'd ever had, and it was impossible to keep them organized. There were just about no days when they were all adjusted and ticking along in good time. And there were many days when not one or two but three or even four were deathly ill, while the nurses were more and more burned out, exhausted, and demoralized.

Except for Mr. Nicks. Mr. Nicks was amazingly stable.

I saw him morning and evening, and gradually, despite his deafness, muteness, and paralysis, I began to understand what Dr. Bee meant by his sweetness. He was always in his chair, polished and shined and groomed by the nurses, when I arrived. He held his head up, he was proud of his mustache, and his eyes were bright. I would sit on his bed. We would look at each other. His one not-roving eye would look at me appreciatively, man to woman. He would give me a smile, raise his eyebrow flirtatiously, and smile some more. Sometimes I would write on my clipboard: "How are you? Any problems?" and show it to him. He would slowly parse out what I'd written. Then he would look at me and shake his head no. Sometimes he even got out, "I'm fine!"

They say that bilateral thalamic strokes can leave a patient looking happy and peaceful while in fact he is having excruciating pain, and that may have been the case with Mr. Nicks. Although, since he could write, frown, and groan, and his choice was "Fine!" and a smile, I think not. He did not seem perturbed by his terrible predicament. He was unmoved, unanguished, with his little smile under his big mustache, and his shiny bright eyes.

I found myself looking forward to our visits, when no one was asking me to undo what God had done, set them on their feet to walk out of the hospital and take up those lives stolen away in the blink of an eye, one fine day, years before.

———

Only once did Mr. Nicks get sick.

It was morning and I was walking around the ward to set my eyes on each patient. Despite the newly instituted Team Communication Board upon which everyone, from doctor to janitor, was supposed to communicate about a patient, and the even-newer electronic Twenty-four Hour Report, I still found it best to make rounds. Those who knew the patients best—the nurses and nursing assistants who actually took care of them—were too busy to write everything down, and besides, there is nothing like seeing, smelling, hearing a patient. It is a CT scan and an MRI and twenty lab tests rolled into one. Often I discovered a patient missing in action, sent over in the middle of the night and admitted to the County Hospital without the Team Communication Board and the electronic Twenty-four Hour Report knowing about it, and sometimes I found a patient who should have been sent over and hadn't been.

So it was this morning. As I reached Bed Number 19, I saw that Mr. Nicks was not in his usual place, dressed, and shaved, bright-eyed in his wheelchair. He was in bed. The nursing assistant hurried over to tell me he was sick. He hadn't eaten breakfast, and he was warm.

What was his temperature? I asked.

It was 96.2.

I sighed. Ever since the advent of the electronic thermometer, it had become impossible to get an accurate temperature. The idea had been that the electronic thermometer would be more efficient than the mercury thermometer—they were supposed to be more accurate, and thus to save time and money. But that calculus hadn't taken account of the fact that the electronic thermometers had to be recalibrated every week, and if they weren't—and they never were—their results would range from 92 degrees Fahrenheit to 99.8, no matter how feverish the patient. For a while I compensated by carrying my own mercury thermometer, but eventually I went back to the eighteenth century and used the pulse rate and warmth of the skin to diagnose a fever.

I went over to Mr. Nicks's bed and looked at him. His eyes were closed, his face was flushed, and his skin was warm and clammy. I shook him and his eyes opened and then closed again. I took his pulse. It was 70. A pulse of 70 is normal and sounds good, but it wasn't good if Mr. Nicks had a fever. Then his pulse should be more like 100. Not 70. In the context of a fever, 70 was slow and meant something was up.

"What's his blood pressure?"

The nursing assistant read from her notes. "It's eighty over we-couldn't-get-a-reading-with-the-machine, Dr. S."

No one had mentioned that on the Team Communication Board or in the Twenty-four Hour Report, and they should have. Because that was a very low blood pressure. It meant that Mr. Nicks was very sick. If he had an infection, the infection was in his blood, poisoning his system, secreting chemicals that relaxed his blood vessels and prevented his brain and heart from getting the oxygen they needed. From a blood pressure of 80, things could go downhill fast—to 60, to 0. Plus, with that pressure his pulse should have been 120, so something was interfering with his heart's ability to beat. He would have to go the County Hospital, and we had an hour or so to do that before he crashed. In the meantime, he needed an IV, fluids, oxygen, and close attention.

I looked up. There were no nurses to be seen, just a social worker talking to a patient. The nurses were at a mandatory meeting.

"Can you get a nurse?" I asked the nursing assistant. "Have her start an IV and oxygen, and call an ambulance. I'll stay with Mr. Nicks."

She hurried down the ward and as I waited, I jiggled Mr. Nicks every minute or so, so that his eyes opened and his pulse and blood pressure went up. Finally a nurse appeared with oxygen, and she began working on the IV. But she was having problems getting it started. And Mr. Nicks was getting worse. His blood pressure was down to 60.

Lupe, the social worker, came over.

"Dr. S, should I call a Code Blue?"

It was a good question. A few years before I would have said, Of course. I would have wanted the Code Blue team to come running, fill up the ward with doctors, with nurses who could start an IV in a flash, with a code cart containing every medication I might need.

Now I hesitated.

Mr. Nicks didn't need a code at that moment; his heart was still beating and I knew we had time. Not much time—in an hour he would need a code. But not right then. So I had some time to fuss with him, to use the tricks I'd learned, and in the meditative silence of the quiet ward. If Lupe called a Code Blue, panic, noise, and disarray would arrive, and a routinized Code Blue would go into effect. A scribe would take notes, analyzed afterward by the Code Blue Analysis Committee, which wouldn't, however, pay attention to whether Mr. Nicks survived or not. It would pay attention to whether the Established Code Protocol had been followed. And therein lay the rub.

Because over the previous two decades, cardiac resuscitation had been routinized. In the hope of getting better results than the 3 percent survival that was the norm, consultants began analyzing codes and experimenting in the lab. A nationwide standardized protocol was formulated, and health-care providers were expected to follow it religiously. We had to take an exam every two years, and if we deviated from the protocol, we failed. Meanwhile, the consultants continued to analyze and experiment, and they changed their protocol every few years, without, however, acknowledging that what had been dogma two years before was now heresy. If you used what had been required the year before but was now banned, you would be questioned. Like any religion, the Code Blue religion demanded faith in its infallibility.

I knew because I kept my Code Blue protocols over the three decades of my practice. Bicarbonate is crucial! was followed by Bicarbonate is never to be used! Electric shocks are to be staggered! Shocks are to be maximized and immediate! Shocks are not to be given! The same with administering calcium (Yes! No! Sometimes!), magnesium, amiodarone, lidocaine, and even chest compressions. Yet, in my experience, these treatments and others were all effective—sometimes, with certain patients.

And though I wasn't sure which collection of yeses and nos this year's Code Blue team would bring to Mr. Nicks's bedside, I knew it wouldn't be what I would do. I'd run many codes, and like most doctors with this experience of what does and doesn't work, I had a personal collection of tricks. And as I stood by Mr. Nicks and waited for the IV to go in, and got the report of the next blood pressure, which was 50, the trick I wanted to use was a medication that is never used in a Code.

It's called Narcan—naloxone. It was formulated as an antidote to morphine and heroin overdose and is their opposite. It counteracts what morphine and heroin do, which is slow down the respiration and pulse, and lower the blood pressure. Naloxone reverses those effects. So when we suspect an overdose of narcotics, we give Narcan.

But over the years I'd noticed that Narcan works even when there is no narcotic overdose. If I gave Narcan when a patient coded, sometimes that would do the trick: the patient's respiration would pick up, his pulse and blood pressure increase, even if there were no narcotics involved. Research in rats showed that it worked well at reversing the dying process. But it wasn't part of the Code Blue protocol.

That it works is not perhaps so surprising, because we know that the body produces its own narcotics called endorphins—endogenous morphine. And after I'd seen Narcan work in other near-death patients who were found not to have any exogenous morphine on board, I began to wonder if our natural endorphins were specifically for the end of life and even the proximate cause of near-death experiences. The tunnel, the white light, the dead family members, the euphoria.

So as I waited for the ambulance, and Mr. Nicks's blood pressure, pulse, and respiration fell, I knew that if Lupe called a Code Blue, he would get everything but Narcan, and I wanted to give him Narcan, even though I was pretty sure he didn't have an overdose. I asked the nurse to get me a vial while I waited by his bed. Mr. Nicks was dying. His blood pressure was down to 50; he was hardly breathing, his pulse was weak, and he was unresponsive. But the ambulance would arrive shortly, his IV was going, his oxygen was on, and he was alive. Lupe had stopped what she was doing and was watching from the end of the ward.

The Narcan arrived and I injected it and put my fingers on Mr. Nicks's pulse. Immediately his pulse strengthened and quickened. A few seconds later, his body shuddered, he took a deep breath and opened his eyes. His blood pressure came up to 90, and then the ambulance arrived, the paramedics transferred him to a gurney and trundled him out.

Lupe came over and watched as out the door they went. Then she turned to me. She didn't say anything, but she raised her eyebrows and I raised mine back.

The whole time Mr. Nicks was at the County Hospital, I worried. What had I done? He was deaf, mute, and paralyzed, and he was never going to get better. Had I done the right thing?

True, I had followed the Advanced Life Directives so laboriously obtained by Dr. Bee, and not just their letter but their intent. Because if I had just followed their letter, he might have been dead. He wouldn't have gotten Narcan but whatever the Code Blue du jour was giving—which at the time was epinephrine, and might have worked or not.

But I had tried something that worked. And not only worked but worked in a horrible way, blocking the chemicals that Nature created to make passing from life to death gorgeous, splendid.

We know Narcan is horrible because that's what our drug abusers tell us after—their pupils pinpointed, heart rate down to 22, respiratory rate at one breath per minute—we give them Narcan and reverse their overdosed state. It's the worst feeling in the world, they tell me, just as heroin is the best feeling in the world.

The best? I've asked them.

Yes.

Better than orgasm?

Way better. Heroin's rush is an orgasm not just of body and mind but of the whole universe exploding. And Narcan is Hell. The worst. Going from best to worst.

I thought about the French calling the orgasm *la petite mort*—the little death. If orgasm is a little death, doesn't that make Death itself—the Big Orgasm?

It wouldn't be surprising. It's easy to imagine that at that last moment, that very last moment of life, all the body's chemicals are released at once—endorphins and cortisol and epinephrine and dopamine and serotonin and chemicals we don't yet know about—so that the moment of death is superb, splendid, the best. That's what *The Tibetan Book of the Dead* tells us, and that's what those near-death experiences imply—and why not? If, as the Bible says, "Love is strong as Death," then Death is strong as Love. You don't have to be a believer to believe that. You can be as atheistic as you want, and still look forward to a final moment of ecstasy, of knowing that it's perfect, it's superb, it's as it should be.

And I had taken that blissful experience from Mr. Nicks. I wondered how he felt about that and how he felt about being alive. I wondered, even though I had followed his own directives, would he have given me the same directives if he had known what he was directing me to do?

Mr. Nicks turned out to have urosepsis, a poisoning of the blood by bacteria from the bladder, and thanks to the ICU and the antibiotics of Fast Medicine, he came back a week later. I was nervous. Would he have deteriorated and lost the little he could still do? Would he be angry? What should I do the next time?

The ambulance drivers rolled him in. He was sitting upright on the gurney. The County Hospital had done a good job. He was clean and dressed, his mustache had been clipped, his hair trimmed.

I went over and looked at him with my question in my eyes.

He looked back at me with his right eye, while his left eye went eastward. Slowly a smile formed on his face, and slowly he raised his one good hand. Thumbs-up!

Really? I looked at him closely.

He looked me in the eyes as forcefully as he could, and nodded. He was happy to be alive, and glad that I'd followed his directives and used that Narcan, and that he wasn't dead. In spite of all his disabilities, in spite of everything he couldn't do, Life was still rich, still worth living.

Mr. Nicks would be my last lesson, or, more accurately, the first lesson in my next class.

With him and his non–Code Blue, I finally felt satisfied. I had passed the Test. He was my sign of having come through one grade of mastership and entered the next. With him I'd had to practice Fast Medicine and Slow Medicine not sequentially but all at once: slowly practicing Fast Medicine—the blood pressure, the pulse, the Narcan—and fastly practicing Slow Medicine—scanning him as a whole, placing him against his environment. I'd had to find Fast in the midst of Slow and Slow in the midst of Fast, all the while staying in the place where Fast and Slow come together.

Mr. Nicks's thumbs-up! meant something over and something new. I had achieved a new level of mastery. What that new level was, was mysterious, and that mystery beckoned. It had something to do with Slow, with the set and style, the place that Slow brings you to in yourself—and also requires.

In the meantime, things were getting worse and worse in the hospital, harder and harder. Doctors were leaving, in disgust and in frustration, retiring or getting laid off. The number of nurses was halved, the hardworking certified nursing assistants had their salaries cut, while more and more administrators were hired to oversee us.

There were more and more forms—five-page forms, ten-page forms, even twenty-page forms!—so many forms that the charts would explode from them, and Medical Records would have to take out the doctors' notes to make room. There were more and more meetings, and the patients were sicker and sicker because, abandoned and ignored, they were at the bottom of the pecking order, no matter what Marketing said about Community and how the Patient Came First.

I was determined to stay, nonetheless.

And then came the day of my never-to-be-completed physical exam of Mr. Raoul Rivero.

I didn't know much about Mr. Rivero, and, as time would tell, I would never learn very much about him, though I did try.

He was tall and pleasant, fifty-two years old, with good manners and big square glasses. He was originally from El Salvador, without papers and, therefore, without health insurance. Twelve years before, he'd been hit by a car while walking across the street. His neck had been broken and his spinal cord injured. He was taken to the County Hospital, where the fracture was repaired and he had acute rehabilitation, but then he'd been sent to us because he was still mostly paralyzed. He continued to work on his own rehabilitation, however, and had improved to the point where he was able to stand in the parallel bars and do his exercises, using his arms to carry him back and forth on his still-weak legs ten or twelve rounds. I would see him every morning at the bars when I came in. He was determined to walk again, to be independent, and so every time a team of discharge planners tried to discharge him, he refused, politely but clearly. He would leave the hospital when he could walk again, he told them.

He spoke only Spanish but my clinic Spanish served us well enough, and he always gave me the sense that he, unlike most of our patients, was middle-class, a businessman from a good Salvadoran family.

It had been time for his annual physical exam for quite a while, and though by then they were out of fashion, both Administration and I were pushing me to do one. Administration, because the hospital was always a decade behind fashion, and in the newly installed computer program, an alert for Mr. R's annual physical exam came up at every use. I, because I always found those annual physical exams useful, despite the evidence-based studies demonstrating their uselessness. I was ever amazed by just how much the physical exam could reveal. Not only did it give me a thorough knowledge of the patient's body going forward, not only did it reinforce confidence in me as a doctor, but often it uncovered some unexpected contributing reason for a patient's disability. After all, Mr. R could have another reason for his persistent weakness. He could have developed something else—a thyroid problem, a kidney problem, a cancer, which I would want to know about.

I'd never yet had an occasion to examine him, and on this particular day I was determined to do so. I would get to know him, finally. So I came in early, saw my other patients, and then had two hours for Mr. Rivero's exam.

It was satisfying. I was examining him the way Dr. Gurushantih had taught me, from stem to stern, top to bottom, head to toe. I was right in the middle, examining his abdomen, when the Head Nurse, now in a bureaucratic coup renamed "Nurse Manager," came in.

"Sorry to bother you, Dr. S, but Philip is here for his ten o'clock meeting."

Darn. I'd forgotten. Philip the Pharmacist. We'd agreed to meet at ten a.m. the first Wednesday of each month to go over the new pharmacy demands that were required by all the newest regulations. Starting the year before, every month I would get a stack of printouts concerning my patients, with the pharmacy's suggestions about which medications I should use and even about which lab tests I should order. The suggestions were almost always trivial—to change one antihypertensive to another of the same class, or to vary the timing of a medication—but occasionally they were completely wrongheaded. Such as "Dear Health-Care Provider. Your patient, Mr. X, has anemia and is not on iron. Please consider checking his hematocrit and starting him on iron."

The computer program, polite and well programmed as it was, did not understand that Mr. X was terminal and had requested no further blood tests, or that iron in any case would be the wrong treatment for his chronic anemia. As the health-care provider, however, I was supposed to respond to the computer's demands by explaining in the chart why I was not ordering its suggested follow-up test for anemia or prescribing iron. Which I would do. But the computer program would not change, and so the next month the same polite but implicitly threatening request would appear, and I would have to write yet another paragraph of explanation. It was beyond time-wasting.

So Philip and I had agreed to meet monthly to go over all those requests in person, thus clearing them permanently. And here he was. And there went my time with Mr. Rivero. Would I ever be able to finish his exam? That ward, with its severely ill collection of patients, and the times, with their ever-changing regulations and requirements, were a rising tsunami about to submerge me.

I was torn. I wanted to finish with Mr. Rivero but Philip was hot-tempered, thin-skinned, and intractable. He would be angry if I didn't appear and he would report me on some form or another.

So I left Mr. Rivero's room.

I found Philip sitting at the nursing station with all the charts piled up and the printouts next to the charts. He did not smile when he saw me.

I sat down and he opened the first chart and the first printout and asked me to change my order from one stool softener to another. I began to write. But I was also thinking how I would never be able to complete Mr. R's exam.

I rewrote the order, and Philip handed me the next chart. I was to rewrite this order because I had used the nongeneric name of the medica-tion, and there was a new regulation that only the generic form be used. I rewrote that order, thinking how there was no one left in Administra-tion who would notice or care whether I completed Mr. R's exam or not. I could just leave it half done. From the computer and administra-tive point of view, Mr. R would have had his required annual exam, and whether it was missing half or not would matter to no one except me. Perhaps I could just—leave it half done. Dictate half, write half. I wouldn't have to lie, I could just write what I'd done, and QED.

And at that very thought, the right half of the page I was reading became wiggly. I blinked. The wiggliness did not go away. It spread.

Philip handed me the third chart. I was to change this order from "twice daily" to every twelve hours.

What difference did that make? I asked. It was a long-acting medication.

Regulations, he replied.

My vision was going on the right. So I was having either a retinal detachment or a stroke. If it was a retinal detachment in my right eye, then the vision in my left eye would be fine. If it was a stroke, the vision in both eyes would be wiggly.

I closed my right eye, and the vision in my left eye was wiggly. It wasn't a retinal detachment. So I was having a stroke, apparently. I stood up.

Philip waited as I walked to the back of the nursing station. My vision was getting worse. Soon, I knew, I would be falling to the ground uncon-scious, with a grand mal seizure. The Head Nurse—Nurse Manager—would call an ambulance, I would be taken to the University Hospital and wake up in a month, paralyzed on my right side, unable to speak.

I left the ward and walked down the long hall into the doctors' cavern, where we'd been exiled when Administration took over all our little doctor offices. I went over to my desk and sat down. I took some deep slow breaths and waited for what would come next.

SIXTEEN

A Slow Medicine Manifesto

And then my vision stopped getting worse. After about fifteen minutes, it began to clear. It wasn't a stroke after all but what Oliver Sacks hypothesized had caused Hildegard's visions—a visual migraine. How poetic. After half an hour, I stood up, let the on-call physician know I was leaving, and went home.

I'd always wondered when my last day would be. That was it. I did come back to go over my patients and sign off my charts, but I never did complete Mr. Rivero's physical exam.

And so my years at the almshouse came to an end.

I began looking around for yet another place where I could be the doctor I'd learned to be. It was harder to find than I thought.

There was an old piece of the County Hospital, now turned into its Urgent Care Clinic. A 1915 brick building with carved cornices, carpeted lobby, and tiled fireplace, it had elevators that didn't work but windows that did. A ramshackle but tended Hildegardian garden surrounded it, with rosemary, digitalis, lavender, sage, and mint. In the waiting room, patients took a number and sat down in folding chairs, and the exam rooms had scratched brass fixtures and porcelain sinks. There were lots of sick patients with no place else to go, and I thought I'd be happy there for a while, until its number also came up. But I was wrong, I realized on my second day, when I saw the Case of the Earworms, which I'll tell you about sometime.

Next I went on an interview for a position at the Old Mission, taking care of its retired nuns. That building, too, was old and brick, and nestled among green hills. Quiet, out-of-the-way. It smelled right, it looked right, and I could so imagine practicing medicine there. It reminded me of Ms. Lloyd's clinic. There was the big table in the middle, the little examining rooms against the walls.

The medical director who interviewed me was smart, practical, and knew all about Hildegard. He had even walked the pilgrimage to Santiago de Compostela. We talked for an hour, and then he sighed and said, "Now let me show you where you'll be spending most of your time."

I looked around. Yes, something was missing. The place smelled right and looked right, but there were no doctors, no nurses, and during the hour I'd been there, no patients. Where was everybody?

I followed him down a long, low-ceilinged corridor, and with a sad flourish, he opened the door on the left.

I saw a big room, dimly lit, with rows of computers and health-care providers sitting at them, tapping and squinting.

The medical director knew, even before he showed that room to me, that I wouldn't take that job, and I didn't. Why would I want to spend all my time in front of a computer screen?

After that, I kind of gave up. I missed seeing patients, and I did keep my ear out, but every time I heard of a promising place, someplace forgotten, with windows that opened, funky examining tables, RNs with furrowed faces, and the smell of paper, alcohol, bandages, and human beings, there was always that long corridor to that room with all those blinking screens, waiting for me to come and take care of them instead of patients.

Instead, I began writing *God's Hotel*.

In the meantime, Carlo Petrini's Slow Food Movement had taken off. It grew. There were Slow Food demonstrations, meetings, and colloquia in Italy, an International Slow Food Conference in Paris. Slow Food organizations sprang up in Germany, England, and more than a dozen other countries. The movement released a "Slow Food Manifesto," proclaiming that food is the joy and heart of life, and that it is wrong to commodify, industrialize, and destroy its essence, which is Taste. What is right is to enjoy food and bow to its producers, acknowledging the pleasure and community that, as the Buddhists say, come to us from the work of many people and the suffering of many forms of life.

The Slow Food Movement's message came to America's shores and also spread. You could even say it came back to our shores like an echo, and resonated with the maturing strains of the organic food movement, the hippie culture, and the political concerns from which it was derived. Small is good, all politics is local—that Aquarian Revolution I had seen brewing so long ago. "Slow" itself took off, became a theme—slow parenting, slow living, slow sex.

Counter culture, literally and in fact.

So by the time I began thinking about what should come next for me, there it was, to hand. An opposing principle, an opposite pole to the ever more powerful hegemony of efficiency in healthcare. Slow, as in Slow Medicine.

I wasn't the only doctor to put "Slow" and "Medicine" together. There were others making that connection, at just the same time. It was a natural connection to make, especially when you think about the ancient Galenic dictum that "all food is medicine." First in Italy and then in the United States, a light went on—if we need Slow Food, we really need Slow Medicine. There were different emphases and different interpretations. Some used Slow Medicine to mean mainly taking time, holding back, not rushing in to do something to a patient. For others Slow Medicine meant a careful reading of the evidence, a Dr. Greg kind of skepticism, a focus on not "overdiagnosing," on not "overtreating." In Italy, Slow Medicine emphasized the social and political implications of a measured, fair, and just system of care.

For me, "Slow Medicine" meant and means a way of understanding the medicine I've seen, learned, and grown to love. It signifies a Way—a way of seeing, doing, and being.

It is a way of seeing, that gardener's way I learned from Hildegard, of stepping back and seeing the patient in the context of his environment. And asking, What is in the way of the patient's own healing power of Nature? And then removing what's in the way.

It is a way of doing, which is slow, methodical, and step-by-step. Although that "Slow" is not temporally slow. Rather, its pace is slow, dispassionate, unhurried, and unrushed. So you can be "Slow" in the midst of Fast, as I learned from Mr. Nicks. Measured. Tempered.

And it is a way of being. That "just sitting" with the patient I finally learned at Laguna Honda, a person-to-person "just sitting," a mutual healing.

It is not a Way that excludes "Fast" or the Way of Fast. It does not reject seeing the body as a machine and being a good mechanic, who traces the source of his patient's suffering to its origin, who might even take things apart, repair and replace. Nor does it reject the tools of the fantastic medical progress I have witnessed in my life as a physician. Rather, it is a Way that incorporates Slow and Fast, the Way of the Gardener and the Way of the Mechanic, that sees these two Ways as tools in its little black bag and uses the right tool for the job. It is a solid Way built on excellence—of method, of knowledge and experience, of hard work. But also on the personal, the individual, and the face-to-face.

After *God's Hotel* was published, and I started to get the thousands of letters and give the hundreds of talks it led to, I began to realize that Slow Medicine itself was turning into a movement, a Slow Medicine Movement. It was most like the organic food movement, which, too, had started small, in the orchards and fields of those farmers I first heard about at the Neumanns'—and whose products are now in Walmart and Safeway and all of our pantries. In the same way, Slow Medicine has been developing as a grassroots movement, growing underground, with experiments popping up here and there. In England, a Slow Medicine Clinic; in Berkeley, a Slow Medicine Project, with a whole set of new ideas waiting to be put into practice. For instance, there can be a Slow Medicine Fellowship for medical students to learn what it means to be slow. We can allow for Slow Medicine beds in our hospitals so that doctors have enough time to find out what is really wrong with a patient, and patients have enough time to heal. We can even create a new kind of consult service—a Slow Medicine consult service!—for those complex patients—like my father—where we know we've missed something crucial but nobody has the time to find out exactly what.

Most thrilling of all is that this Slow movement in general—and the Slow Medicine Movement in specific—is setting up a kind of opposite pole to the techno-body, the virtual, data-producing, data-consuming body that Marketing promotes, which is a fine approach to the body and to health as long as you're not sick. Once you're sick, however, as I learned at Turnaround, once you become a patient—vulnerable, scared, passive—then you need a doctor, a real doctor-person—calm, authoritative, wise. And since all of us, even the youngest, healthiest, fiercest hacker will, in the end, be in that place—which to discover we must travel to—we all need a system that incorporates both: the virtual and the real, the digital and the analog, the Fast and the Slow. And I believe we will have it.

We're not there yet, however. In the meantime, there is likely to be an increasing polarization of the Twos, as the Two Fishes of Pisces swim in opposite directions and their connection grows ever more taut. More polarization of left/right, man/woman, black/white, fast/slow, the exaggeration that occurs as one Age is ending but another is not yet arrived. There was one final roar of the raging Arian Ram in Rome as the Age of Pisces was appearing; there was one last charge of the Taurean Bull as the Arian Age came on. We can expect the same as the Age of Aquarius arrives—Jung's collision of the opposites, an *enantiodromia*, where top becomes bottom, inside becomes outside, where what was rejected becomes accepted.

We're already seeing this in medicine: a reversal, an unconscious acceptance of the previously rejected, a thinking of the formerly unthinkable. Suddenly we realize: DNA is not, as dogma has had it for thousands of exam questions, the only carrier of genetic material. RNA can also carry genetic material, and so can—unthinkable!—proteins, and what else? Darwin's long-dismissed opponent, Lamarck, is now acknowledged to have been not wrong in his idea that the environment can lead to permanent genetic change. Even germs—so long the enemy to be defeated in our war against disease—are all of a sudden not to be always and everywhere destroyed. In the newly discovered "microbiome," germs are now our allies, our helpers, even our necessities, even our "us."

The stone that the builders rejected becomes the cornerstone.

Jung foresaw a coming of the Age of Aquarius, which would be an age of integrating the unconscious with the conscious into a wholeness. And now the Age of Aquarius is upon us, and it is time to put together the opposites; in medicine, Fast Medicine and Slow Medicine, the Way of the Mechanic and the Way of the Gardener. But not together as in a pot. Rather, as two different ways of acting, which, as I saw with Mr. Nicks, contain each other. After all, sometimes even a plant is best treated as a machine, and a machine as a plant. The gardener who eyes the dead leaves and branches and cuts them off; the mechanic who fusses and fiddles and chucks his machine under the chin.

The solution is that opposites do not unite but contain one another— Slow has Fast within it and Fast has Slow, and *that* Slow has Fast. It's the recursiveness of these two Ways, that they can contain each other ad infinitum, which creates wholeness out of difference, which allows us to find the Slow in the Fast, the Fast in the Slow, while staying unmoved and calm at that single point of Self.

Acknowledgments

I never would have written this book without the thousands of readers of *God's Hotel* whose e-mails and letters so often included a story, point of view, or question. They made it clear that the Way of Slow Medicine needed exposition.

Thanks to all who invited me to speak and so gave me a forum not only for speaking but also for listening, where I could learn what was really happening across the country as medicine was becoming healthcare. Particularly inspiring was Dr. Charles Hatem of Harvard's Mount Auburn Hospital, a forty-year veteran of medical student teaching. He let me understand how dedicated the Academy is to making sure the best doctors are formed. Also Dan Church, President of Bastyr University, for his insight and presence. And E. Craig Moody, head of the Mark Twain Literary Club of San Francisco, for insisting that my writing must have had a long gestation. His challenge forced me to rediscover the writing I'd done for decades, and Beryl, Dr. Langley, and Mr. Sunshine.

For inspiration that it is possible to change things: Bernie Lown, Laura Marshall-Andrews, David Meltzer, Rosanne Haggerty.

My Slow Medicine friends and colleagues, including the late Dennis McCullough, Ladd Bauer, Katy Butler, Michael Hochman, Pieter Cohen, José Carlos Campos Velho, and Giorgio Bert.

The Department of Medicine and the Department of Anthropology, History and Social Medicine at the University of California, San

Francisco, especially its Chair, Sharon Kaufman, for her support and so many wonderful discussions. Rani Marx, Susan Ivey, and Jim Kahn for their determination to make Slow Medicine real.

My parents, still perspicacious and lively after nine decades. My sisters—three variations on a theme of strength, intelligence, wit, and ambition. Special thanks to Robert Leathers for his warm hospitality and his deep dedication to engagement and inquiry.

My first readers: Patricia Wick, always ready to read a new piece, incisive, calm, enthusiastic; Eleanor Sweet, such a good writer herself; and Rebecca Moore, inspiring in her own work, and always there to cheer me on and remind me why I was writing this book.

Many friends, among whom: David Kleber, Diane Ross-Glazer, Melanie MacMitchell. Rosalind Pierce, Susan McGreivy, Meg Newman, Ann Fricker, Theresa Berta, Grace Dammann, Eric Jamison, September Williams, and Professors George and Phyllis Brown, models of the engaged academic.

The coming generation, warm, open, thoughtful, but also ambitious and optimistic—especially Jeff Leathers, Ed Leathers, Allison Wick, and Katherine Wick.

The passing generation with its revolutionary values and its vision of a City on the Hill.

Without my agent, Mary Evans, this book would never have come into existence. Thoughtful, critical, and passionate, she always has my best interest and the best interest of the book in mind.

Rebecca Saletan, my wonderful editor. She read every line twice, fought for the best wording, and insisted I write this book and also apply for a Guggenheim.

The Guggenheim Foundation for awarding me a Guggenheim Fellowship. It couldn't have come at a better time for giving me the encouragement and conviction I needed to start this big project.

Everyone at Riverhead, so dedicated to making beautiful and intelligent books. Special thanks to publisher Geoff Kloske, Katie Freeman and Claire McGinnis in publicity, art director Helen Yentus, and Anna Jardine in copyediting.

My partner, Jenny, for our lively, intellectually stimulating home full of flowers and friends. And our Bernese Mountain Dog, Tallit, who teaches me each day that dogs don't have to live as long as people because they enjoy and cherish every hour.

Last, I want to acknowledge the grace and kindness of the late Oliver Sacks, model of the physician-writer, the doctor-philosopher, who exemplified the modesty that comes from wisdom.

Notes

INTRODUCTION: MEDICINE WITHOUT A SOUL

1 *seizures are terrifying, though mostly they don't hurt you:* For two sources that review the topic, see J. Engel, Jr., "So What Can We Conclude—Do Seizures Damage the Brain?" *Progress in Brain Research* 135 (2002), 509–512, and Johanna Palmio, "Seizure-Related Neuronal Injury: A Study of Neuron-Specific Enolase, S-100b Protein and Tau Protein," doctoral dissertation, University of Tampere, 2009. Both conclude that there is no evidence to show that a single seizure injures the brain.

CHAPTER ONE. ON THE CUSP OF AQUARIUS

18 *called the "Great Year":* Understanding what it was like to live in a geocentric cosmos is critical for understanding the point of view of most premodern cultures. That cosmos, where the earth is the center and movement happens around it, explains why the medical systems of China, India, and the West are so similar to one another, though not identical. I only understood it when I spent one moonless night outside with an astrolabe—the medieval computational device constructed on the notion of the geocentric cosmos. With it I watched the stars move overhead and saw how they didn't just rise and set but also rotated around the fixed point of the North Star. For a brilliant introduction to the implications of this concept, see Giorgio de Santillana and Hertha von Deckend, *Hamlet's Mill: An Essay Investigating the Origins of Human Knowledge and Its Transmission Through Myth* (Jaffrey, NH: David R. Godine, 1977).

22 *the unconscious, the* Unbewusste*:* For Jung's definitions of these archetypes, see the glossary at the end of *Memories, Dreams, Reflections*, where his editor, Aniela Jaffé, pulls together quotations from his various works to illustrate his concepts. Here, these are my understandings of them. Jung separates the contents of that *Unbewusste* into three kinds of unconscious: the *Unbekannte*, the unknown in the sense of either once known but no longer known, i.e., forgotten, unremembered, repressed, blocked; the not-yet-known; and the unknowable. I have not, however, been able to find anywhere my inference from his *anima* and *animus* definitions: that to the extent we have an *anima*, an internal woman, that internal woman must have an internal *animus*, and that there is a recursiveness to this model. See Carl Jung, *Memories, Dreams, Reflections*, ed. Aniela Jaffé, trans. Richard and Clara Winston (New York: Vintage Books, 1989).

22 **The motive force for change was** enantiodromia: Jung wrote that he took the concept from Heraclitus, but it seems he got the word *enantiodromia* from a later compilation of Heraclitus's work by Joannes Stobaeus. It translates as the "running of the opposites," and the idea is that whatever is too extreme flips into its opposite; there is a basic balancing function in the mind, a compensatory function. We see this all the time: The violent homophobe turns gay; the atheist becomes a religious zealot. I understand this natural balance, this pendulum, as demonstrating that inside every extreme is a kernel of its own opposite: inside every liberal is a conservative; inside every conservative is a liberal. For a good essay on Jung and *enantiodromia*, see Sue Mehrtens, "Jung on Enantiodromia: Part 1—Definitions and Examples," Jungian Center for the Spiritual Sciences, http://jungiancenter.org/jung-on-the-enantiodromia-part-1-definitions-and -examples/#_ftn2.

CHAPTER TWO. DR. GURUSHANTIH AND MY NEW WHITE COAT

26 *the creation of medical schools in twelfth-century Paris:* Medical school per se started not in Paris but in Salerno, but my point here is that the making of medicine into a university profession on the level of theology and law happened first in the universities of twelfth-century Paris, which accepted only (male) clerics. See Susan Lawrence, "Medical Education," in William F. Bynum and Roy Porter, eds., *Companion Encyclopedia of the History of Medicine* (New York and London: Routledge, 1997), vol. 2, 1153–1157.

26 *Yet of our school's 120 professors, only two were female:* It is remarkable how long it took women to be admitted to the guild of medicine, considering it was women who naturally did much of the medical care in the premodern world. Brewing and cooking, sewing and gardening, were women's jobs, after all, easily applied to the needs of the body. A study of women in medicine published in my second year revealed pornographic photos in anatomy class, sexual attacks in dark closets, the intimidation of women medical students, and even threats. Perhaps most telling, it was published by the only woman dean in the country under a pseudonym. See Margaret A. Campbell, *"Why Would a Girl Go into Medicine?" Medical Education in the United States: A Guide for Women* (Old Westbury, NY: The Feminist Press, 1973).

29 *"There are three sexes":* The quote from Osler appears in Lilian Welsh, *Reminiscences of Thirty Years in Baltimore* (Baltimore: Norman, Remington, 1925), p. 44. There's a deeper truth to Osler's witticism that links up to Jung's *anima/animus* insight. Perhaps the real "third sex" that women doctors have to learn to be— tough and tender, cool and warm, intimate and objective, doctor and nurse—is, when you come down to it, what all doctors need to learn to be.

CHAPTER THREE. THE MAN WITH A HOLE IN HIS HEAD

41 *perhaps he had multiple myeloma:* Multiple myeloma is a cancer of plasma cells, which are white blood cells in the bone marrow whose job is to make antibodies. The classic symptoms and signs are bone pain, an elevated calcium, neurologic changes, and kidney dysfunction. The neurologic symptoms often include depression, confusion, and weakness from the elevated calcium, and headaches from the increased blood viscosity that results from the plasma cell clones' increased production of a single antibody. The diagnosis is usually made using serum M or urine M spikes, but can also be suggested if lytic lesions are seen on plain X-rays. The diagnosis is confirmed with a bone marrow biopsy. On his skull film, Mr. Harris had the classic "raindrop" or

punched-out appearance. With current treatments, the average survival after diagnosis is seven to eight years. See "Multiple Myeloma," in Dan Longo et al., eds., *Harrison's Principles of Internal Medicine*, 18th ed. (New York: McGraw-Hill Medical, 2013), vol. 1, 936–942.

CHAPTER FOUR. DR. GREG'S 30 PERCENT SOLUTION

54 *One day I pulled out a dusty book from a shelf:* Harold Gillies's *Plastic Surgery of the Face: Based on Selected Cases of War Injuries of the Face Including Burns* (London: Oxford University Press, and Hodder and Stoughton, 1920) can be seen online at https://archive.org/details/plasticsurgeryof00gilluoft.

57 *Every study had a "placebo" set:* The two best studies I've found on the nature of the placebo effect are Henry K. Beecher, "The Powerful Placebo," *JAMA: The Journal of the American Medical Association* 159, no. 17 (December 24, 1955), 1602–1606; and T. J. Kaptchuk and F. G. Miller, "Placebo Effects in Medicine," *The New England Journal of Medicine* 373, no. 1 (July 2, 2015), 8–9. Beecher wrote one of the first reviews of the placebo effect, and makes a brilliant distinction between dummy pills and placebos. "Dummy" pills show the effect of natural healing, while placebo pills also show the effect of the mind on healing. Summing up the results of twenty-three years of trials, he concluded that placebos had an average effectiveness of 35 percent. Sixty years later, Kaptchuk tried to tease out the "natural healing" effect from the psychological effects of placebos in a drug trial where he compared active pills labeled "placebo" with active pills labeled with their chemical names. He concluded that "placebo effects are modest as compared with the impressive results achieved by lifesaving surgery and powerful, well-targeted medications."

CHAPTER FIVE. A SUCCESSFUL PETITION
TO THE SAINT OF IMPOSSIBLE CAUSES

63 *neurofibromatosis—elephant man's disease:* Since Marcela, we've learned a great deal about neurofibromatosis and not just about the disease, but about what the disease tells us about the body. There are two known types; both are caused by mutations in a gene that produces a protein which inhibits the growth of "things." The manifestations of NF1 result from a mutation in or deletion of the NF1 gene. The gene product, "neurofibromin," serves as a tumor suppressor; decreased production of this protein results in the uncontrolled growth of neurofibromas, optic nerve fibromas, gliomas, astrocytomas, meningiomas, etc. Only one NF1 gene of the two everybody has need be deleted or mutated to produce the disease; a more severe phenotype is seen in the subset of patients with a complete gene deletion. The second type of neurofibromatosis, NF2, has a different problem: a mutation in the gene that produces a cytoskeletal protein and leads most of the time to bilateral vestibular schwannomas. For a good summary, see N. P. Hirsch, A. Murphy, and J. J. Radcliffe, "Neurofibromatosis: Clinical Presentations and Anesthetic Implications," *BJA: British Journal of Anaesthesia* 86, no. 4 (2001), 55–64.

63 *And this was a truly terrible diagnosis:* Marcela's plexiform bladder tumor as a presenting sign of neurofibromatosis is a rare manifestation of a rare disease, and at the time was so rare as to be reportable. See, for instance, S. S. Clark, M. M. Marlett, R. F. Prudencio, and T. K. Dasgupta, "Neurofibromatosis of the Bladder in Children: Case Report and Literature Review," *The Journal of Urology* 118, no. 4 (October 1977), 654–656.

68 *But it would be Joey Canaan who would introduce me:* For an article about Joey, see Rip Rense, "Joey Looks Forward to Merry Christmas," *Valley News* (Van Nuys, California), December 12, 1976, 1. The article (here in condensed form) quotes Joey's mother: "'You know, when the doctors told us he was going to die, we lost all hope. But he kept getting better and better. When he came home we were so worried we spent the first month just standing by his bedroom door.'" It goes on to say that "the concern was unwarranted, however, because Joey continued to defy doctors' predictions and recovered so fast that his mother said 'no one can believe it.'" She maintains it was the combined prayers of hundreds of people and a candle lit at the National Shrine of St. Jude in Chicago that kept her son from succumbing to injuries that could have taken the life of any hardy adult."

70 *Saint Jude, the patron saint of impossible causes:* The website of the National Shrine of Saint Jude informs us: "The National Shrine of St. Jude and the St. Jude League bring together hundreds of thousands [of] devotees in a community of prayer and hope to our patron saint. We invite you to join us and send your prayers to St. Jude as he has proven to be a beacon of hope to those facing seemingly impossible trials and tribulations." http://www.shrineofstjude.org/site/PageServer?pagename=ssj_homepage.

CHAPTER SIX. THE MANTLE OF HIPPOCRATES

81 *Dr. Grace and his six children:* On Dr. Grace, see Keri Brenner, "Nicholas Grace: He Lived Life to the Fullest," *Healdsburg Patch* (California), October 9, 2011, and Clark Mason, "Nicholas Grace, Healdsburg Physician, Dies at 77," *The Press Democrat* (Santa Rosa, California), October 6, 2011.

82 *"It's the Mantle of Hippocrates":* Along Aquarian-revolution lines, there was a movement at the time, and still is today, to not take the classic Hippocratic Oath because of its sexism and guildism. Instead, each medical school should create its own version, with the result that over the years the Hippocratic Oath devolved first into a promise, then into an intention, a desire, a wish, a try-my-best, and is far less compelling than an oath. Perhaps this is one of those times that the wisdom of tradition should outweigh the opinions of the moment.

CHAPTER SEVEN. THREE PROPHETS, NO WHALE

88 *why the Freudians called him schizophrenic:* Not only did the Freudians say that Jung was schizophrenic; he said it himself during a period in his life after he'd broken away from Freud. He heard voices, saw visions, and thought he might be "menaced by a psychosis" or "doing a schizophrenia." See Carl Jung, *The Red Book: Liber Novus* (New York: W. W. Norton, 2009), p. 202.

90 *I was reading not only Freud and Adler . . . but also the anti-psychiatrists:* I had a problem with the concept of mental illness, which was why I liked the anti-psychiatrists Ronald Laing and Thomas Szasz, who both emphasized the subjectivity of the diagnosis. Laing suggested it was a fever of the mind and, like a fever, had a purpose; Szasz's point of view was that schizophrenia was the packaging of unsocial attitudes and actions into a disease model. What bothered me the most was that, even if psychosis turned out to be a brain disease, that didn't imply that what my patients saw by means of their disease was false. Just because we know the mechanism of something doesn't mean we know its significance.

91 *Was George Johnston as Mr. Sunshine sick or well?* The disease of schizophrenia was defined in the 1870s by the psychiatrist Eugen Bleuler, Jung's mentor. At the time,

medicine was moving from thinking of illness as an imbalance of humors to thinking of it as made up of specific entities, and Bleuler wanted to understand madness, too, as a specific disease. So he moved into his hospital and lived with his patients for twelve years, taking notes of what they did and said. What most impressed him about their disease was that it was as if the usual connections among their mental functions (*phrenia*) had been cut (*schizo*)—so he coined the term *schizophrenia*. By that he meant, therefore, not a "split mind" but a loose mind. Indeed, as I would see during that year, the schizophrenic was all over the place, his speech tangential and circumstantial, and his metaphors not symbolic but real. The paranoia and hallucinations were secondary. For more on Bleuler, see Henri F. Ellenberger, *The Discovery of the Unconscious: The History and Evolution of Dynamic Psychiatry* (New York: Basic Books, 1970), 285–289.

102 *He wasn't paranoid or hallucinating, tangential or circumstantial:* As psychiatric interns we learned how to interview and examine patients from *The Psychiatric Interview in Clinical Practice*, by Roger A. MacKinnon and Robert Michels (Philadelphia: W. B. Saunders, 1971). It was a very different exam from DeGowin and DeGowin's— no touching. The disease we were trying to diagnose was in the mind, not in the brain; psychosis was, by definition, a "thought disease." Despite the lack of touching, though, the psychiatric examination had a lot to it. At its best, it was what I would later call "slow." It was about watching and seeing. How did the patient enter the consultation room? Stiffly? Restlessly? Like a wild animal on soft feet, smelling around the corner, ears up? Cocking his head to better hear his voices? Was his speech rapid and all over the place—pressured, tangential, and circumstantial? Was he excited? Or slow-moving? Ponderous, heavy? From that exam, we would then make our diagnosis, usually of "psychosis," and within that category, of schizophrenia, mania, or depression. Once in a while the diagnosis would not be psychosis but a severe neurosis, hysteria, or drugs, or even someone who just wanted a bed for the night, although, I discovered, psychosis is surprisingly hard to fake.

102 *As the* DSM *said:* We learned how to diagnose patients from the *DSM-II, The Diagnostic and Statistical Manual of Mental Disorders: Second Edition.* That edition was 168 pages; today's, the fifth, is 624 pages and includes a lot more of the eccentricities of humanity as psychiatric diagnoses. It was, or tried to be, the *Harrison's* of psychiatry. Just as *Harrison's Principles of Internal Medicine* categorized disease into types and causes—infectious, cancerous, autoimmune—so the *DSM* divided mental diseases into psychoses, neuroses, and personality disorders, and then subdivided psychoses into schizophrenia, mania, and depression, and psychosis unspecified. Like *Harrison's*, too, it differentiated these diseases using their symptoms and signs—"symptoms" being what the patient said, and "signs" being what the doctor found on exam. And yet, somehow, it was fundamentally different from *Harrison's* because it was so much more subjective. For instance, if the patient said he or she heard voices, that was "hallucinating," a symptom of psychosis, unless there were, in fact, voices, in which case, it wasn't a symptom of psychosis. This turned out not to be as farfetched as it sounds. One of our attendings, Dr. Coleman, told us about a patient he had diagnosed with schizophrenia on the basis of his hearing voices. He'd treated the patient unsuccessfully for months, until one day he realized that the patient was in truth hearing voices—the metal fillings in his teeth were picking up radio broadcasts. He wasn't schizophrenic after all, and Dr. Coleman sent him to the dentist. The same for "delusions"—of being followed or commanded by the FBI or the KGB. This was a symptom of psychosis, unless the patient was in fact being followed or commanded by the FBI or the KGB. So it was subjective and the psychiatrist had to be a kind of detective.

CHAPTER EIGHT. VISITING DAY AT THE HENHOUSE

120 *Kathy, however, trusted my physical exam and left for Mr. Schumer's:* Why did Kathy go and I did not? I wasn't as confident as Kathy that my diagnosis was right, and my attitude was—I did my best. I fulfilled my physician duty. And if I'd come in the next morning, and Mr. Schumer was dead of his dissecting aneurism, I would have been regretful, but I don't think I would have felt guilty, because I did not conceive the idea of going to his house. It wasn't in my repertoire. At the time, and even today, I see the two callings of doctor and nurse as different. Doctors diagnose and treat; nurses look after. But are they different? It depends on how you interpret *treat.* There are doctors who conclude that *treating* means treating the root cause of the disease, and they become politicians, social reformers, and revolutionaries. Kathy broadened my thinking of what it meant to be satisfied with my treatment, and though I never did take on her idea of a calling, I did think more deeply afterward about where my responsibility to a patient ended.

CHAPTER NINE. A SLOW MEDICINE CLINIC BEFORE ITS TIME

131 *Everything I'd learned in medical school did exist, no matter how rare:* Just to give an idea, a partial list of what I saw in that clinic includes parasites: *Giardia lamblia, Trichuris trichiura, Dientamoeba fragilis, Strongyloides stercoralis,* pinworm, hookworm, *Clonorchis sinensis, Ascaris lumbricoides, Entamoeba histolytica, Taenia solium,* and *Hymenolepsis nana.* Infectious diseases included tuberculosis and dengue, Chaga's disease, malaria, histoplasmosis, coccidioidomycosis; chlamydia, syphilis, gonorrhea, *Lymphogranuloma venereum,* and Reiter's disease. Genetic diseases included Fragile X, Turner's syndrome, Wilson's disease, and testicular feminization. Benign tumors included pituitary tumors and cerebellopontine angle tumors, and malignant tumors included breast cancer, uterine cancer, vulvar and cervical cancer, gallbladder cancer, malignant histiocytosis, sarcoma, and acute leukemia.

131 *So I loved practicing medicine in that little clinic:* I was the only one to leave. Dr. Meryl worked at the little clinic until she retired decades later, having ushered many babies through infancy to college; Nurse Lloyd got the clinic through many a crisis, attempted closing, and changes in payment systems, until she, too, retired. Melinda stayed through the AIDS epidemic, and Becky is still there.

131 *It was so simple, and its simplicity was its strength:* Much later I would practice in a similar clinic, which would have three times as many staff to do the same thing—fourteen people, not counting the doctors—in order to deal with all the marketing and quality assurance, economy and efficiency that would, in the meantime, arrive.

132 *They were consultants the county had hired:* I would find out later that the consultants were from National Medical Enterprises Inc. (NME), whose future would exemplify how Medicine was turned into Healthcare. It was founded by three lawyers after Medicare and Medicaid were established and they realized that, with the federal government involved, money could be made in the hospital business. So NME began buying up hospitals—acute hospitals, rehabilitation hospitals, and long-term care hospitals—and running them like factories, with inflows and outflows of patients producing revenue and a strict control of costs. Our county was one of its early near-successes. NME persuaded the Head of the County Hospital to sell the county's ancient Poor Farm to it, which it then promptly closed and sold. Then the Head of the Hospital outsourced his own job to NME, in a contract where they, the lawyers, would manage the hospital. After that he himself went to work for NME. Eventually its name was changed to Tenet Healthcare, and it is now a publicly traded multibillion-dollar

health-care company. For these details and more, see for example http://www.bmartin.cc/dissent/documents/health/nme_founders.html (last updated July 2007).

133 *I thought about the new plan:* For details of the eventual plan, see "The Health Plan of San Mateo" at http://www.plsinfo.org/healthysmc/22/finances_work.html. "In a unique risk-sharing arrangement, Primary Care Providers and hospitals are divided into five physician-hospital risk pools. . . . Each PCP must associate with one of these five pools. . . . Primary Care Providers are paid a monthly capitation based on the age, sex, and eligibility category of each of their enrollees. These payments are currently subject to a 10% withhold. . . . Primary Care Providers are at risk for primary care, specialty care, and pharmaceuticals. . . . Surplus payments are shared among the PCPs, hospitals, and HPSM. Primary Care Physicians and hospitals are protected by contractual stop-loss provisions. Specialist physicians and other providers are reimbursed on a fee-for-service basis and are not at risk." In this new system, one would do best to be a specialist and continue to get paid for one's work.

137 *It was a cure and I was amazed:* Could Lee's cure have been a placebo effect? Or the power of natural healing? Perhaps. In one study that looked at the placebo effect on asthma, patients reported substantial improvement not only with inhaled albuterol (50 percent improvement) but also with inhaled placebo (45 percent) and with sham acupuncture (46 percent). In contrast, the improvement reported with no intervention was only 21 percent, which is still considerable when you think about it. See M. E. Wechsler et al., "Active Albuterol or Placebo, Sham Acupuncture, or No Intervention in Asthma," *The New England Journal of Medicine* 365 (2011), 119–126.

CHAPTER TEN. PASSING THE POINT OF NO RETURN

142 *get so little sleep:* The eventual decrease in residency hours was triggered by the death of a patient that was ascribed to a sleep-deprived resident, and the idea was to prevent any such further deaths. It has had variable effects, not all of them good. The most obvious not-good effect is that the 116 hours a week of training I unwillingly received could only be approximated if the residency was extended by at least one year, and it wasn't. So medical residents now are shortchanged of one-third of their experience. The second not-good effect has been that residents are now treated like shift workers, required to come to the hospital at a specified time and leave at a specified time, regardless of how sick their patients are. So they take care for ten hours of someone else's admitted patient, and have to leave to other doctors their own patients. It is a built-in discontinuity of care and prevents the life-changing experience I would get when I tended Mrs. C minute by minute, hour by hour, and day by day for sixty-three days.

INTERMISSION: IN WHICH FAST MEDICINE AND SLOW MEDICINE COME TOGETHER

157 *Hapsburg chin:* I did not have a photo of Mr. English, nor did he and I exchange names. But it was easy to find a photo online of Sir Geoffrey Gould Briggs, Chief Magistrate of Hong Kong, who retired in 1979 and died in 1993 and spent most of his life in the Far East, and there he is with his Hapsburg chin.

167 *the distinction between apprentice and journeyman:* The apprentice was contracted to a master for a certain number of years, lived in the master's house, and received food, lodging, and training. After his contract was fulfilled, he became a journeyman and was then paid for his work but could not yet employ others. So you could say that at this point I had just fulfilled my apprenticeship and was about to be a journeyman. For

more, see Georges Renard, *Guilds in the Middle Ages*, ed. G. D. H. Cole, trans. Dorothy Terry (1918; New York: Augustus M. Kelley, 1968).

CHAPTER ELEVEN. TURNAROUND

169 *The storm was AIDS, although that wasn't its first name:* For an overview of the history of AIDS, see the article at the AVERT website, http://www.avert.org/professionals/history-hiv-aids/overview. What I portray here, however, is not the canonical view but the developing story as it looked from the eye of the storm, when we didn't know what would happen or what the cause would turn out to be. My very first case was a young man with diffuse lymphadenopathy who showed up at the little clinic and I could not figure out what he had. Then I read the first reports—M. S. Gottlieb et al., "Pneumocystis Pneumonia—Los Angeles," *Morbidity and Mortality Weekly Report* 30, no. 21 (June 5, 1981), 1–3 (https://www.cdc.gov/mmwr/preview/mmwrhtml/june_5.htm), and A. E. Friedman-Kien, "Disseminated Kaposi's Sarcoma Syndrome in Young Homosexual Men," *Journal of the American Academy of Dermatology* 5, no. 4 (October 1981), 468–471. And when a second young man came in with the same diffuse lymphadenopathy, I did recognize it as this something new and sent him up to the City for diagnosis. How we began to think about it once we knew it was a new disease is well described in Lawrence K. Altman, "New Homosexual Disorder Worries Health Officials," *The New York Times*, May 11, 1982, Science section.

170 *a fine pink rash:* Two years after Dr. Dobbins told me about that rash, a description of it was published; see M. H. Rustin, C. M. Ridley, M. D. Smith, and M.C. Kelsey, "The Acute Exanthem Associated with Seroconversion to Human T-Cell Lymphotropic Virus III in a Homosexual Man," *Journal of Infection* 12, no. 2 (March 1986), 161–163.

170 *a new virus they named "human immunodeficiency virus":* HIV—human immunodeficiency virus—has taught us a tremendous amount about the body, much of it overturning previous dogma. It is a retrovirus—"retro" because its instruction code is RNA, which has to be translated "back" into DNA by the cell it infects. Its RNA is wrapped in an envelope, and sticking out of the envelope are structures that allow the virus to land on and attach to the CD4 "helper cell" of our immune system. This triggers a structural change that invaginates the cell membrane and takes the virus into the cell. The virus then uses its own enzyme, DNA reverse transcriptase, to translate its RNA into DNA, which then integrates itself into the CD4 cell's own DNA. And there it stays inactive until something *else* happens—we don't yet know what—and the cell starts to transcribe that HIV DNA into RNA. That RNA then engineers the creation of the necessary proteins and enzymes to make a complete virion, which self-assembles and then buds off from the cell. The cell weakens, deteriorates, and dies; our CD4 population begins to decline, and at a level of around 200, the kind of cancers and infections they protect against—Kaposi's sarcoma, lymphomas, pneumocystis pneumonia, everything I saw during those years—begin to appear. But what keeps the HIV DNA quiescent for so long, and what starts it reproducing, is not yet known.

171 *we began to see a flood of cases:* I derive my approximation from a *New York Times* estimate that 40 percent of the single men in San Francisco at the time were gay ("San Francisco Survey Finds 40% of Single Men to Be Homosexual," November 23, 1984) and from a report that, by 1984, 50 percent of the gay men in San Francisco were HIV-positive, up from 25 percent in 1982 (W. Winkelstein, Jr., et al., "The San Francisco Men's Health Study: III. Reduction in Human Immunodeficiency Virus Transmission

Among Homosexual/Bisexual Men, 1982–86," *American Journal of Public Health* 77, no. 6 [June 1987], 685–689).

180 *In Hebrew there is a concept called teshuvah:* In answer to my question about how *teshuvah* relates to the English "turning," Alan Elbaum, a Geniza scholar, writes (in personal correspondence): "The BDB (authoritative biblical Hebrew dictionary) defines the root שוב as 'turn back, return,' and *teshuvah* as 'returning to God,' an extension of the original physical meaning."

182 *I hadn't grasped the archetype of Physician:* Is there a Jungian archetype of Physician? There is something numinous about what is demanded of us physicians, and I finally found it in Jung's essay "The Phenomenology of the Spirit in Fairy Tales," where he describes the archetype of the "Wise Old Man." The Wise Old Man appears as a doctor sometimes in dreams and represents knowledge, insight, cleverness, and intuition, as well as "moral qualities such as goodwill and a readiness to help which make his 'spiritual' character sufficiently plain." Jung touches upon the most important aspect of this archetype, I believe, when he emphasizes that the Wise Old Man is "a life-bringer as well as a death-dealer. . . . Indeed the old man has a wicked aspect too, much as the primitive medicine-man is a healer and helper and also the dreaded concocter of poisons." The ambiguous aspect of this archetype that the doctor plays into is why there is so much ambivalence around physicians and why such overwhelming, impossible qualities are expected of us—the virtues of mother, father, saint. He who can cure can also cause; he who can heal can also afflict; he who can save a life can also take a life. So the archetype of the Doctor is the archetype of the Magician. As patients, we must be certain it is used correctly, hence our impossible list of virtues. See Carl Jung, *Archetypes and the Collective Unconscious,* trans. R. F. C. Hull, vol. 9 of *The Collected Works of C. G. Jung* (Princeton, NJ: Princeton University Press, 1981), 207–255; quoted from 222, 227.

182 *As long as there is sickness:* The hospital, too, is an archetype, I believe, embodying the ancient tradition of the City on the Hill and the monastery—a community dedicated to the common good.

CHAPTER TWELVE. A CRAFT, A SCIENCE, AND AN ART

184 *students become masters themselves:* The classic description of the medieval guild system is by Georges Renard, and it describes the guild of medicine well: "Industry was carried on under a system of enterprise at once public and private, associative and individual. The unit of production was the workshop of the individual master-craftsman; but the craftsman held his position as a master only by virtue of full membership in his Craft Guild. He was not free to adopt any methods of production or any scale of production he might choose; he was subjected to an elaborate regulation of both the quantity and the quality of his products, of the price which he should charge to the consumer, and of his relations to his journeymen and apprentices. He worked within a clearly defined code of rules which had the object at once of safeguarding the independence, equality and prosperity of the craftsmen, of keeping broad the highway of promotion from apprentice to journeyman and from journeyman to master, and also of preserving the integrity and well-being of the craft by guarding the consumer against exploitation and shoddy goods." It sounds worthwhile even today. See Georges Renard, *Guilds in the Middle Ages,* ed. G. D. H. Cole, trans. Dorothy Terry (1918; New York: Augustus M. Kelley, 1968), 9.

188 *"it builds up in the blood and causes hepatic coma":* The two articles Dr. Rose would have read are Robert K. Kerhan, Jr., et al., "Portal-Systemic Encephalopathy Due to a Congenital Portocaval Shunt," *American Journal of Roentgenology* 139 (November

1982), 1013–1015, and N. H. Raskin, D. Bredesen, W. K. Ehrenfeld, and R. K. Kerlan, "Periodic Confusion Caused by Congenital Extrahepatic Portacaval Shunt," *Neurology* 34, no. 5 (May 1984), 666–669. Since then a number of other cases have been reported; for instance, see Ali Sobia, Alan H. Stolpen, and Warren N. Schmidt, "Portosystemic Encephalopathy Due to Meso-iliac Shunt in a Patient Without Cirrhosis," *Journal of Clinical Gastroenterology* 44, no. 5 (May–June 2010), 381–383, and Yuta Kasagi et al., "Non-Cirrhotic Portal-Systemic Encephalopathy Caused by Enlargement of a Splenorenal Shunt After Pancreaticoduodenectomy for Locally Advanced Duodenal Cancer: Report of a Case," *Surgery Today* 44, no. 8 (August 2014), 1573–1576. Kasagi and colleagues write: "In patients with a portal-systemic shunt, neurotoxic substances such as ammonia flow directly into the systemic circulation and may cause encephalopathy without liver cirrhosis" (1575).

189 *I crossed them off my list:* On toxins as a cause of hyperammonemia: there was, for instance, "methionine analogue produced in wheat flour during the agenizing process in vogue between 1920 and 1950. . . . It improves the flour but converts some of the methionine to methionine sulfoximine. . . . It produces running fits, canine hysteria and fright disease." Irwin H. Krakoff, "Effect of Methionine Sulfoximine in Man," *Clinical Pharmacology and Therapeutics* 2, no. 5 (September 1961), 599–604. Was this effect due to ammonia? Yes, it was. "Methionine sulfoximine (MSO), an inhibitor of glutamine synthetase, produced disinhibition about 3 hours after administration; at this time cerebral ammonia was increased to 290% of normal, glutamine was unchanged. . . . [It] produces an endogenous ammonia intoxication which: (i) decreases the amount of exogenous ammonia required to affect cortical postsynaptic inhibitions; and (ii) eventually becomes sufficiently severe to disturb cortical inhibitory neuronal interactions by itself." See W. A. Raabe and G. R. Onstad, "Ammonia and Methionine Sulfoximine Intoxication," *Brain Research* 242, no. 2 (June 24, 1982), 291–298; quoted from the abstract.

190 *I kept it on my list but moved it lower:* On poison as a cause of hyperammonemia: "Systemic poisoning induced by the parenteral administration of ammonium salts or rese, e.g., purified jackbean urease, has been extensively studied in laboratory animals. . . . It produces a self-perpetuating cyclic release . . . [that] results in a sustained 24–49 hours elevation of blood ammonia . . . but the survivors made a complete, rapid recovery." I used this quotation for my Grand Rounds but cannot find the source.

190 *episodes of confusion, psychosis, or seizures:* I did worry that Mrs. MM's 40 percent OCT activity might have been related to her terminal state when we got the biopsy. The liver mitochondria start to deteriorate after death, although the biopsy was obtained before the respirator was turned off. Late-onset patients, as she was, have residual OCT enzyme activity ranging from 26 to 74 percent of normal control values, so Mrs. MM's values fit the diagnosis exactly. For a summary article, see Uta Lichter-Konecki et al., "Ornithine Transcarbamylase Deficiency," *Gene Reviews*, posted August 29, 2013, last updated April 14, 2016, http://www.ncbi.nlm.nih.gov/books/NBK154378.

190 *diagnosis of schizophrenia:* The biggest hint that Mrs. MM's basic problem was not liver failure but an OCT deficiency was her level of ammonia, which rose from 320 to 460 to 644 to 710 to 818 in one day. Today we know that anything over 500 is suggestive or even diagnostic of a urea cycle disorder. On issues of the laboratory testing of ammonia, see the Evidence-Based Medicine Consult at http://www.ebmconsult.com/articles/lab-test-ammonia-nh3-level.

191 *"She's brain-dead and I'm ordering":* The Harvard criteria for brain death were put together in 1968. They include unreceptivity and unresponsiveness; no movement or breathing; no reflexes, often proved with cold calorics—by irrigating the tympanic membranes with ice-cold water to produce a reflex brainstem deviation of the eyes. If

negative they imply brainstem death. A flat electroencephalogram is confirmatory. They are fulfilled only if the body temperature is greater than thirty-two degrees centigrade and in the absence of central nervous system (CNS) depressants. See "A Definition of Irreversible Coma: Report of the Ad Hoc Committee of the Harvard Medical School to Examine the Definition of Brain Death," *JAMA: The Journal of the American Medical Association* 205, no. 6 (August 5, 1968), 337–340.

194 *and the elevator doors opened:* Could Mr. Danska's response to carotid sinus massage have been that he was having supraventricular tachycardia (SVT) and not ventricular tachycardia (v-tach)? For an article showing that termination of a tachycardia by carotid sinus massage does not necessarily prove its supraventricular origin, see D. S. Hess et al., "Termination of Ventricular Tachycardia by Carotid Sinus Massage," *Circulation* 65, no. 3 (March 1982), 627–633.

198 *The report of Mrs. Mather's OTC test:* The results of Mrs. MM's biopsy took four weeks to come back. And during those four weeks there was a coincidence that puzzled me as much as her results enlightened me. The article "The Natural History of Symptomatic Partial Ornithine Transcarbamylase Deficiency" was published, and the date of its publication was the day I was in the library, researching Mrs. MM. It describes what I had hypothesized: women with a partial OCT deficiency can have episodes of confusion and end up with a psychiatric diagnosis. See P. C. Rowe, S. L. Newman, and S. W. Brusilow, "Natural History of Symptomatic Partial Ornithine Transcarbamylase Deficiency," *The New England Journal of Medicine* 314, no. 9 (February 1986), 541–547. My biggest question about Mrs. MM, though, has always been what would have happened if we had dialyzed her. I've kept track of the literature over the years. There have been patients with OCT deficiency, comatose from elevated ammonia levels, who woke up after dialysis. So . . . perhaps.

CHAPTER THIRTEEN. UPSTAIRS, DOWNSTAIRS

201 *the founding of the "Slow Food Movement":* Carlo Petrini wrote his history of coming to the idea of Slow Food in *Slow Food: The Case for Taste,* trans. William McCuaig (New York: Columbia University Press, 2003; originally published as *Slow Food: Le ragioni del gusto* in 2001). In his *In Praise of Slowness: Challenging the Cult of Speed* (New York: HarperSanFrancisco, 2004), Carl Honoré describes different aspects of Slow—Slow Sex, Slow Parenting, and Slow Health Care—although not what we have come to call Slow Medicine.

211 *the phrase "health-care provider":* The logical result of this definition is the economists' demand that health-care providers "wisely steward society's resources," as they like to say. It sounds good in theory, but in practice, less so. It implies that health-care providers have different ethical values from those of physicians. As health-care providers we apply principles of public health to our consumers, not the Hippocratic principles where the individual doctor-patient relationship is paramount. For example, we should direct resources to ensure that everyone has his immunizations and not that some particular patient who neglected to get a tetanus shot and now has tetanus gets the best, perhaps expensive, treatment. As a citizen, I can see their point, but as a patient I have to know that I, and not the budget, am the main concern of my doctor.

213 *his results, which were normal:* In specific, the tests I ordered for Ric were a CBC and chemistries, an HIV test, a VDRL, thyroid tests, ANA, RA, SPEP, Lyme titers, brucellosis titers, B12, folate, and lead level. They were all normal or negative. The CT of Ric's back was also negative. The article I found at the time was G. C. Román, "Retrovirus-Associated Myelopathies," *Archives of Neurology* 44, no. 6 (June 1987),

659–663. On the possible success of Ric's treatment, see a later review by Unsong Oh and Steven Jacobson, "Treatment of HTLV-I-Associated Myelopathy / Tropical Spastic Paraparesis: Towards Rational Targeted Therapy," *Neurology Clinics* 26, no. 3 (August 2008), 781–797.

223 *demanding that the Board remove itself and hold new elections:* The petition read: "We the undersigned demand that the present Board of Directors be removed, and a new Board elected or appointed to replace it, which will be composed of at least 51% patients as is set forth in the by-laws. The current Board (none of whom are patients of the clinic) has turned a deaf ear to the doctors' concerns about patient care and closed their eyes to the needs of the staff. They have remained dumb when confronted with obvious abuses of the system by the present executive director. No minor concessions will change the downhill course. We must have people on the Board who care enough to take an active interest in the way it is run and who will refuse to let it deteriorate through their own inaction or cowardice."

223 *all four of my tires had been slashed:* I would love to tell you the eventual outcome in detail, but I still have a car with four tires.

A SHORT PAUSE TO RECAPITULATE, OR THE CRACK IN THE COSMIC EGG

227 *The Crack in the Cosmic Egg:* I took this part of the chapter title from Joseph Chilton Pearce, *The Crack in the Cosmic Egg: New Constructs of Mind and Reality* (New York: Julian Press, 1971). For more on Hildegard as a medical practitioner, see Victoria Sweet, "Hildegard of Bingen and the Greening of Medieval Medicine," *Bulletin of the History of Medicine* 73, no. 3 (Fall 1999), 381–403.

231 *the chicken or the egg:* For more on this vision, see chapter 6 of my book *Rooted in the Earth, Rooted in the Sky: Hildegard of Bingen and Premodern Medicine*, ed. Francis G. Gentry (New York and London: Routledge, 2006). For more on the sheela-na-gig tradition, see Barbara Freitag, *Sheela-na-gigs: Unraveling an Enigma* (London: Routledge, 2004).

CHAPTER FOURTEEN. THE FORCE THAT THROUGH THE GREEN FUSE DRIVES THE FLOWER

233 *The Force That Through the Green Fuse Drives the Flower:* The title comes from Dylan Thomas.

247 *And what can I do to fortify it? Viriditas* led me on a merry dance. For an extensive discussion, see chapter 5 in my *Rooted in the Earth, Rooted in the Sky* (cited in the notes to the previous chapter). The connections between green and grow, green and the greenback, green and modern ecology, the Red Revolution and the Green Revolution, are fascinating to trace. Suffice it to say that the person who brought us "green" as an image of ecology was a French monk, Peter Maurin, who knew of *viriditas* from Albertus Magnus, another monk who wrote on plants in the century after Hildegard.

248 *they got better and better:* For a much more detailed exploration of the politics and personalities, see my book *God's Hotel: A Doctor, a Hospital, and a Pilgrimage to the Heart of Medicine* (New York: Riverhead Books, 2012).

CHAPTER FIFTEEN. NOTHING IS BETTER THAN LIFE

249 *Nothing Is Better Than Life:* I take this idea from Masanobu Fukuoka's *The One-Straw Revolution: An Introduction to Natural Farming*, trans. Larry Kor (New York: New

York Review of Books, 2009). Fukuoka phrases the thought as "There is nowhere better than this world." His concepts about gardening and being a gardener parallel those I have developed here about doctoring and being a doctor.

256 *cardiac resuscitation had been routinized:* On resuscitation, Saint Augustine says it best: "Who considers the works of God, by which he orders and makes orderly the whole world, and is not stunned and completely silenced by the miracles? . . . The dead resurrect, people are amazed; daily they are born, and no one is amazed. And if we consider, it is more amazing to make something which was not, than to resuscitate what was." My condensation is from the 1873 translation by the Reverends John Gibb and James Innes of Tractate VIII, Chapter II, section 1, of Saint Augustine, *Homilies on the Gospel of John* (John 2:1–4), at the Christian Classics Ethereal Library website, https://www.ccel.org/ccel/schaff/npnf107.iii.ix.html.

CHAPTER SIXTEEN. A SLOW MEDICINE MANIFESTO

267 *Slow, as in Slow Medicine:* For a history of Slow Medicine, see J. Ladd Bauer, "Slow Medicine," *Journal of Alternative and Complementary Medicine* 14, no. 8 (November 2008), 891–892. For Slow Medicine in Italy, see Giorgio Bert, Andrea Gardini, and Silvana Quadrino, *Slow Medicine: Perché una medicina sobria, rispettosa e giusta è possible* (Milan: Sperling & Kupfer, 2013). As for evidence that giving time back to doctors actually can save money, see David O. Meltzer and Gregory W. Ruhnke, "Redesigning Care for Patients at Increased Hospitalization Risk," *Health Affairs* 33, no. 5 (2014), 770–777.